The Complete
Diabetes Prevention Plan

The Complete Diabetes Prevention Plan

A GUIDE TO UNDERSTANDING THE EMERGING
EPIDEMIC OF PREDIABETES AND HALTING ITS
PROGRESSION TO DIABETES

Sandra Woodruff, M.S., R.D., L.D./N.

Christopher D. Saudek, M.D.

AVERY ■ A MEMBER OF PENGUIN GROUP (USA) INC. ■ NEW YORK

a member of
Penguin Group (USA) Inc.
375 Hudson Street
New York, NY 10014
www.penguin.com

Library of Congress Cataloging-in-Publication Data

Woodruff, Sandra L.
The complete diabetes prevention plan : a guide to understanding
the emerging epidemic of prediabetes and halting its progression
to diabetes / Sandra Woodruff, Christopher Saudek.
p.   cm.
Includes bibliographical references and index.
ISBN 1-58333-183-2
1. Prediabetic state—Popular works.   2. Diabetes—Popular works.
3. Diabetes—Prevention—Popular works.   I. Saudek, Christopher D.
II. Title.
RC660.4.W66   2004   2003062979
616.4'6205—dc22

Printed in the United States of America
10   9   8   7   6   5   4   3   2   1

This book is printed on acid-free paper. ∞

Book design by Meighan Cavanaugh

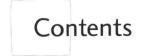

Contents

The Complete
Diabetes Prevention Plan

Introduction

It's no secret that type 2 diabetes is quickly becoming the biggest epidemic of our time. In fact, the number of adults with diabetes worldwide will more than double over the next twenty years. Even more alarming is the number of children who are developing a disease that was once called "adult-onset" diabetes.

What's behind this disturbing trend, and how can you tell if *you're* destined for diabetes? More important, how can you avoid becoming another statistic in the diabetes epidemic? That's what *The Complete Diabetes Prevention Plan* is all about.

As you will see, type 2 diabetes is not inevitable. There are steps you can take to stop it in its tracks—before it becomes irreversible. Many people can even turn back the clock and return their blood glucose levels to the normal range.

The first part of *The Complete Diabetes Prevention Plan* explains how you can go from "normal" to developing diabetes without even knowing it. You will learn about the silent, early stages of diabetes and the newly coined condition, "prediabetes," that already affects millions of Americans. You will also learn about exciting new research that absolutely proves that most cases of type 2 diabetes *can* be prevented by some very simple lifestyle changes.

Part 2 puts principles into practice. Here you will find the latest information on the best foods and dietary strategies for preventing diabetes and for managing prediabetic conditions, such as insulin resistance and the metabolic syndrome. *The Complete Diabetes Prevention Plan* will help you master the practical aspects of transforming your diet by providing a wealth of tips for meal planning, dining out, grocery shopping, cooking, and much more.

Is weight loss part of your diabetes prevention plan? If so, should you cut fat, carbs, or calories? *The Complete Diabetes Prevention Plan* highlights the pros and cons of popular weight-loss diets and offers scientifically sound advice for tipping the scales in your favor. You will learn how to choose foods and plan meals that keep you feeling full and satisfied while you safely lose weight. You will also discover why one "diet" does not fit all, and how a variety of weight loss approaches can help you shed pounds.

What about exercise? Everyone can benefit from being physically active, but as you will see, people who are at risk for diabetes have even more to gain from being active. In chapter 7 you will discover the tremendous benefits of this simple and inexpensive diabetes prevention therapy. You will also find simple, doable strategies that prove that exercise need not be grueling or overly time-consuming to be highly effective.

The remainder of the book provides over 170 delicious, user-friendly recipes that will prove that a diabetes prevention lifestyle can be easy, immensely enjoyable, and special enough to impress family and friends alike. Looking for some new ways to start your day? Chapter 8 presents plenty of ideas, from Ham & Asparagus Omelette and Southwestern Egg Sandwich to Rolled Swedish Pancakes and Frosty Fruit Smoothie. Or perhaps you're looking for some palate-pleasing fare to perk up your next party. Chapter 9 will lead the way with choices like Pesto Party Pizzas and Spicy Spinach & Artichoke Spread. Still other chapters will show you how to make satisfying soups and stews like Italian Wedding Soup, refreshing salads like Asian Chicken Chop Salad, wholesome side dishes like Garlic Smashed New Potatoes, hearty sandwiches like Slimmed-Down Sloppy Joes, comforting pasta dishes like Lazy-day Lasagna, light and tasty entrées like Seared Cajun Chicken, and even something for the sweet tooth like Cherry Fudge Cake and Cinnamon-Peach Crisp.

Through your lifestyle choices you have tremendous power to determine your health, now and in years to come. The information in this book can be instrumental in helping you make the right choices. It is our hope that *The Complete Diabetes Prevention Plan* will prove that a diabetes prevention lifestyle can be enjoyable, practical, and easy to maintain anywhere, anytime, and any place.

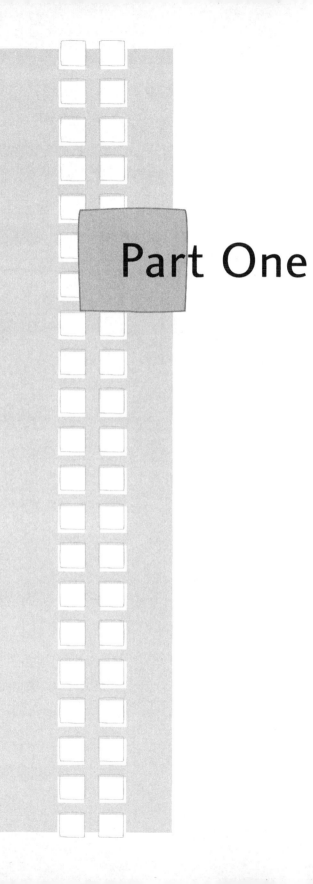

Part One

1. An Epidemic of Major Proportions

Type 2 diabetes—one of the biggest epidemics of our time—currently afflicts 18 million Americans. Three times as common as it was forty years ago, its prevalence matches the dramatic upsurge in the rates of overweight and obesity. But that's just the tip of the iceberg. Even more Americans have a condition known as *prediabetes*—and this may be you. Left unchecked, most will go on to develop full-blown diabetes within about ten years.

The diabetes epidemic is not unique to the United States. In fact, it is rampant around the world. What's behind this alarming trend? And how can you reduce your risk of being affected? This chapter will explain more about diabetes and the newly coined term prediabetes. You will learn the risk factors that set you up for prediabetes or diabetes. And in the following chapters, you will be armed with specific strategies that can dramatically lessen your chance of becoming another statistic in the worldwide epidemic called diabetes.

From "Normal" to Diabetes—What Happens?

Diabetes does not develop overnight. Long before a person has diabetes, the stage is being set. It may be in your genes, and even your development in your mother's womb may have affected your chance of getting diabetes many decades later. But type 2 diabetes is not inevitable—there are things you can do to avoid it. So here are some facts about diabetes and the conditions that lead up to it.

WHAT IS DIABETES?

There are several types of diabetes, but this book is concerned with the most common form, *type 2 diabetes*. Type 2 diabetes makes up about 95 percent of all cases of diabetes and is seen most often in people over thirty-five or so (though, not always, as you will see), in overweight people, and in people who have a history of diabetes in their family.

Put most simply, diabetes is a condition in which the blood glucose (sugar) levels are abnormally high. It is caused by a relative lack of *insulin* (the hormone that keeps blood sugar levels normal) and an impaired ability to process dietary carbohydrate.

Let's look at this in a little more detail. Normally, eating sets off a complex series of events. As food moves from the mouth to the stomach to the intestines, it is systematically broken down (digested) into smaller fragments of carbohydrate, protein, and fats that can be absorbed into the blood. The carbohydrate you eat shows up as sugar (glucose) in the bloodstream, so the blood sugar level rises. At this point, the pancreas normally secretes insulin, which allows the transport of sugar from the blood into the cells. As the sugar moves from the blood into the cells, the blood sugar level comes back down to the level it was before the meal. Inside the cells, sugar can be used for energy right away, or stored for later use.

When someone has diabetes, either the pancreas does not make enough insulin to handle the dietary carbohydrate or the cells do not respond to the insulin (or both). As a result, the sugar stays in the blood instead of entering the cells, while and the cells become starved for energy.

And there's one other important twist: All the sugar in the blood does not come from the carbohydrates you have eaten. The liver makes considerable amounts of sugar, for instance between meals. This sugar also has to be processed under the influence of insulin. So even without eating, if you don't have enough insulin, your blood sugar level can rise.

OTHER NAMES FOR TYPE 2 DIABETES

In the past, type 2 diabetes has been called *adult-onset* diabetes, because it typically occurred in middle-age and older adults. This is no longer the case though, as many children and adolescents who are sedentary and overweight are also developing this disorder. Type 2 diabetes has also been called *non–insulin-dependent* diabetes, which is a misnomer, because some people with type 2 diabetes do need to use insulin. Just to be clear, type 1 diabetes is the form that used to be called juvenile-onset, or insulin-dependent diabetes. It usually comes on in younger, normal-weight people and always requires insulin treatment.

People who do not control their diabetes have chronically elevated blood sugar levels. This "sweetening" of the blood actually causes it to be thicker, like maple syrup. The brain detects this blood as too concentrated and the person becomes thirsty in order to dilute the blood back to a normal concentration. But lacking insulin to help process the blood sugar, the cells are still relatively starved, which contributes to the excessive fatigue that people feel when diabetes is not controlled.

Furthermore, over a number of years, uncontrolled diabetes can also cause serious damage to blood vessels and nerves, leading to complications such as heart disease, loss of vision, kidney failure, amputations, and impotence.

There is no cure for diabetes, although it can certainly be controlled, and the complications can be avoided. The first step in taking care of diabetes is to make some lifestyle changes and, if necessary, take medications, whether pills or insulin by injection. But there is a better way, which is to prevent diabetes before it starts. It is now clear that the progression from prediabetes to diabetes can be stopped, or at least slowed down significantly.

WHAT IS PREDIABETES?

Prediabetes is a condition in which blood glucose levels are higher than normal but not high enough to be considered diabetic. Before people develop full-blown type 2 diabetes, they typically pass through a time when they have prediabetes, although often it is not recognized. Prediabetes has no outward symptoms, because the blood sugar level is not high enough to cause thirst. So you can have it for years without knowing it. However, it's important to identify and treat prediabetes because serious health problems, especially cardiovascular disease, are already progressing at this stage of the game. The National Diabetes Education Program (NDEP) cites three reasons why it's critical to know if you have prediabetes:

■ Having blood glucose levels in the prediabetic range puts a person at a 50 percent higher risk of having a heart attack or stroke.
■ Type 2 diabetes can be delayed or prevented through lifestyle changes.
■ For many people with prediabetes, lifestyle changes can actually *turn back the clock* and return elevated blood glucose levels to the normal range.

Assessing Your Risk

Here are some items that indicate a risk for developing prediabetes and type 2 diabetes. The more risk factors you have—especially if you are overweight—the greater the chance you have one of these conditions. The good news is that many of these risk factors are modifiable, presenting plenty of opportunities to intervene.

RISK FACTOR	COMMENTS
45 years of age or older	As you get older, the likelihood of developing diabetes rises. Approximately 1 out of 5 people age 65 and over have diabetes.
Overweight (BMI greater than 25)	More than 80 percent of people with type 2 diabetes are overweight. The more overweight you are, the higher your risk.
Waist circumference greater than 40 inches (if male) or 35 inches (if female)	Excess fat carried around the stomach is especially linked to insulin resistance and diabetes risk.

RISK FACTOR	COMMENTS
Parent or sibling with diabetes	Having a family history of diabetes raises your risk. The closer the relative, the higher your risk factor.
Ethnic background is African American, American Indian, Asian American, Pacific Islander, or Latino	These ethnic groups are 2 to 2½ times more likely to develop diabetes than Caucasians.
Previously had gestational diabetes, or gave birth to at least one baby weighing more than 9 pounds	Gestational diabetes sometimes occurs during the late stages of pregnancy. It typically goes away after the baby is born, but increases the risk for diabetes in the future.
HDL "good" cholesterol is 35 or lower; or triglyceride level is 150 or higher	Low HDL cholesterol and high triglycerides are both signs that you may not respond to your own insulin normally (a condition known as insulin resistance).
Blood pressure is 140/90 or higher	High blood pressure is often associated with insulin resistance, which underlies most cases of type 2 diabetes.
Exercise less than 3 times a week	Being sedentary impairs the body's cells ability to remove glucose from the blood.

Why and When You Should Be Tested for Prediabetes?

Most people who have prediabetes don't know it. But the damage occurring inside the body is considerable, and left unchecked, prediabetes usually develops into full-blown type 2 diabetes. This is why the National Institutes of Health, the American Diabetes Association, and many health organizations all over the world advise the health-care practitioners to routinely screen patients who are at risk for prediabetes.

If it turns out that you have prediabetes, you should begin taking action right away to reverse the process by using the suggestions outlined in this book and get tested yearly thereafter to be sure you've gotten your levels in check. Even if your test result is normal, if you have any of the risk factors, you should take advantage of the diabetes prevention information here and repeat the test every three years.

Nailing the Diagnosis of Prediabetes

Health-care professionals can use one of two tests to diagnose prediabetes: the fasting plasma glucose (FPG) or the oral glucose tolerance test (OGTT). Both tests measure the body's ability to hold the blood sugar normal. With the FPG, blood sugar is tested first thing in the morning, after an overnight (or an 8-hour) fast. For the OGTT, blood sugar is also tested first thing in the morning after an overnight fast. The person being tested then consumes 75 grams of glucose in a drink and their blood sugar level is tested again two hours later. If the FPG is high (100 to 125 mg/dl), it is called impaired fasting glucose (IFG); if the OGTT is done and the glucose two hours after the sweet drink is 140 to 199 mg/dl, the person has impaired glucose tolerance (IGT).

- Prediabetes is defined as either impaired fasting glucose (IFG) or impaired glucose tolerance (IGT) or both.
- Finding IFG requires only one blood sugar test, easily done in a laboratory. But doing only the fasting blood glucose will miss some people who would have been shown to have prediabetes if the OGTT were done.
- To find IGT, you need the two-hour oral glucose tolerance test.

CRITERIA FOR DIAGNOSING PREDIABETES AND DIABETES		
	FPG TEST RESULT	2-HOUR OGTT RESULT
Normal	70–99 mg/dl	<140 mg/dl
Prediabetes	100–125 mg/dl	140–199 mg/dl
Diabetes	≥126 mg/dl	≥200 mg/dl

Is one test better than the other for diagnosing prediabetes? Not really. Either test is appropriate. The fasting plasma glucose test is much simpler and less expensive, so it is the most widely used, but some people with prediabetes will be missed. The OGTT is less convenient and more expensive, but will pick up everyone with prediabetes. It is recommended that tests for diabetes not be done when a person is sick, for example with an infection or right after surgery, and if positive, it should be confirmed on a different day.

The Causes of Diabetes: Insulin Resistance and Failing Insulin Secretion

Insulin resistance means that the cells of the body don't respond normally to insulin—so they do not take up glucose efficiently in response to insulin. As many as 65 to 70 million Americans have insulin resistance, so it is a very common condition, usually caused by being overweight. To compensate for insulin resistance, a normal pancreas works overtime secreting enough extra insulin to usher glucose into the cells. This extra insulin allows you to maintain normal or near-normal blood sugar levels for some time—thereby staving off type 2 diabetes.

The second piece of the puzzle, the thing that tips a person with insulin resistance into prediabetes or diabetes, is that the pancreas begins to wear out. Over time, it loses the ability to keep putting out enough insulin to overcome the insulin resistance. Then—with the combined insulin resistance and a gradually weakening pancreas—the blood sugar levels start to go up.

So the cause of type 2 diabetes is twofold: the body does not respond to insulin normally (insulin resistance) and the pancreas becomes too exhausted to compensate any longer.

INSULIN RESISTANCE AND THE METABOLIC SYNDROME

For many people, insulin resistance is combined with a cluster of abnormalities even before diabetes occurs. Known by any of several names—*the metabolic syndrome, insulin resistance syndrome,* or *syndrome X,* this group of problems can be very dangerous. The common conditions that cluster together in the metabolic syndrome include high blood pressure, increased blood fats (triglycerides), lower HDL (good) cholesterol, abdominal obesity, above normal blood sugar, an increased tendency for blood clots, and even increased inflammation in the blood vessels. Some researchers think that the abnormally high concentrations of insulin cause this grouping of problems; but whatever the cause, there is no doubt that the metabolic syndrome can triple the risk for heart disease.

How do you know if you have metabolic syndrome? According to the National Institutes of Health, metabolic syndrome is present when someone has three or more of the following indicators:

- Waist measurement greater than 40 inches (102 cm) for men or 35 inches (88 cm) for women
- Blood triglycerides of at least 150 mg/dl
- HDL (good) cholesterol less than 40 mg/dl for men or 50 mg/dl for women
- Blood pressure of at least 135/80 mmHg
- Fasting blood sugar of at least 110 mg/dl

Source: The National Heart Blood and Lung Institute, National Cholesterol Education Program, Third Report of the Expert Panel on Detection, Evaluation, and Treatment of High Blood Cholesterol in Adults (Adult Treatment Panel III). Accessed at *http://www.nhlbi.nih.gov/guidelines/cholesterol/index.htm* 11/21/02.

You will notice that one of the indicators, elevated blood sugar, is also diagnostic of prediabetes. Therefore, some people with the metabolic syndrome already have prediabetes. On the other hand, people who have the metabolic syndrome, but still have normal blood sugar levels, may go on to develop prediabetes if they don't take actions to control their condition.

An estimated *47 million* Americans have the metabolic syndrome, and its rise in prevalence shows no signs of slowing down. These numbers represent the next wave of diabetes and heart disease already in the works. A recent study found that men with the metabolic syndrome were five to nine times more likely to develop diabetes over a four-year period than were men without this condition.

Is there any good news about the metabolic syndrome? Yes. Consider it an early warning sign and an opportunity to turn things around before it's too late. A healthy diet, increased physical activity, and weight loss are the safest, most effective, and preferred means for correcting this metabolic imbalance. The nutrition and exercise guidelines presented throughout this book can help you gain control over metabolic syndrome, as well as prediabetes and type 2 diabetes.

SUMMARIZING THE METABOLIC SYNDROME, PREDIABETES, AND DIABETES

	THE METABOLIC SYNDROME	PREDIABETES	TYPE 2 DIABETES
CONTRIBUTING CAUSES	Genetic predisposition, obesity, poor diet, sedentary lifestyle	Genetic predisposition, obesity, poor diet, sedentary lifestyle	Genetic predisposition, obesity, poor diet, sedentary lifestyle
DIAGNOSTIC CRITERIA	Any 3 of the 5 following signs: • Abdominal obesity • Low HDL (good cholesterol • High triglycerides • High blood pressure • Above normal blood sugar	Fasting blood sugar level of 100 to 125 mg/dl OR Oral glucose tolerance test result of 140–199 mg/dl 2 hours after glucose	Fasting blood sugar level greater than 125 mg/dl OR Oral glucose tolerance test result greater than 199 mg/dl
SYMPTOMS	No overt symptoms	No overt symptoms	If blood glucose is high (generally over 200 mg/dl), increased thirst and urination, increased hunger, sudden weight loss, extreme fatigue, blurred vision, slow healing cuts and bruises, recurrent infections. However, type 2 diabetes may have no symptoms at all. *(continued)*

SUMMARIZING THE METABOLIC SYNDROME, PREDIABETES, AND DIABETES			
	THE METABOLIC SYNDROME	PREDIABETES	TYPE 2 DIABETES
TREATMENT	Healthy diet, exercise, weight loss	Healthy diet, exercise, weight loss	Healthy diet, exercise, and weight loss; many people also need oral medications and insulin to normalize blood sugar levels
COMPLICATIONS	Cardiovascular disease, including heart attack and stroke; left untreated, metabolic syndrome can progress into prediabetes and then type 2 diabetes	Cardiovascular disease, including heart attack and stroke; left untreated, most people with prediabetes will develop full-blown type 2 diabetes within 10 years	Cardiovascular disease, kidney failure, blindness, amputations, impotence

A Dozen Reasons to Prevent Diabetes

- People with diabetes are two to four times more likely to die from heart disease than people without diabetes.
- The risk for stroke is two to four times higher among people with diabetes.
- By the time type 2 diabetes is diagnosed, 50 percent of people already have cardiovascular complications.
- Diabetes is the leading cause of blindness in adults.
- Diabetes is the leading cause of end-stage renal (kidney) disease.

THE DIABETES CRISIS IN CHILDREN

In the past, type 2 diabetes was called *adult-onset* diabetes because it occurred in middle-aged and older adults—and was almost never seen in children. This is no longer the case. Today, more and more children are being diagnosed with type 2 diabetes. And a recent study found that one out of four obese children and one out of five obese adolescents tested already have prediabetes. Furthermore, researchers now estimate that one out of three children born in the year 2000 will develop diabetes within their lifetime. For Hispanic and African American children, the odds are closer to one in two. What's causing this alarming trend?

The rise in childhood diabetes is directly linked to the dramatic upsurge in obesity among children. The link between obesity and diabetes is so strong that researchers have coined the term "diabesity" to refer to obesity-caused type 2 diabetes.

Unless quick action is taken, the health consequences of type 2 diabetes in children will be staggering. A child who contracts diabetes at age ten or twelve may require medications or insulin shots for the rest of their life. Even worse, children with diabetes could develop heart disease, kidney disease, and complications from nerve damage by the time they reach thirty.

What's a parent to do? Encourage children to be more active. Substitute hobbies like sports, dance, and outdoor play for computer and television time. Plan active family outings such as hiking, biking, skating, and swimming instead of going to a movie or out to dinner. Limit the amount of junk food that comes into the home and offer healthful meals and snacks. Above all, set a good example by eating moderately and being physically active.

If your child is overweight, be sure to consult with your pediatrician and a registered dietitian to evaluate causes of the weight problem, address any medical complications, and find lifestyle solutions that will work for your family.

■ Up to 70 percent of people with diabetes have nervous system damage, which can cause lack of sensation or pain in the feet and hands, difficulty with digesting food, and other problems.

■ Diabetes is a leading cause of lower-extremity amputations.

■ Diabetes is a leading cause of impotence.

■ People with diabetes are more likely to have periodontal (gum) disease than are people without diabetes.

■ Poorly controlled diabetes prior to and during pregnancy can cause birth defects and spontaneous abortions, and can result in excessively large babies, posing a health risk to the mother and the child.

■ Uncontrolled diabetes can lead to potentially fatal biochemical imbalances, such as diabetic ketoacidosis and coma.

■ People with diabetes are more susceptible to infections and many types of illnesses, including pneumonia and influenza. Once they become ill, they are more likely to die than people who do not have diabetes.

In summary, prediabetes is the stage between normal and diabetes, and even before prediabetes may come the metabolic syndrome. You can evaluate your own risk and, with

PREDIABETES AND MEMORY LOSS

Need another reason to adopt a diabetes prevention lifestyle? Keeping your blood sugar under control may be a defense against memory loss. Researchers have long known that people with diabetes have an increased risk for memory problems because high blood sugar levels damage blood vessels and nerves that supply the brain and other organs.

Researchers now believe that memory loss may be prevalent in the prediabetes stage as well. A recent study found that people with impaired glucose tolerance had a higher risk of memory loss and shrinkage of the part of the brain that controls learning and memory. The good news is the same simple lifestyle changes that can halt the development of diabetes—dropping a few pounds and being more physically active—could also help your mind stay sharp for many years to come.

your health-care professional, you can find out if you have prediabetes. If so, there are actions you can take to stop it in its tracks. The remaining chapters of this book will help you implement these life-saving strategies. People with the metabolic syndrome, prediabetes, or type 2 diabetes can all benefit from the guidelines for good nutrition and physical activity presented in this book.

2. STOPPING DIABETES IN ITS TRACKS

The dramatic rise in diabetes prevalence is a recent phenomenon, and, we repeatedly emphasize, it is very, very closely tied to the increase in obesity. There is no doubt that heredity also plays a role, and a strong family history of diabetes is a big risk factor for your getting it. But gene pools change very slowly, and the explosion of diabetes is occurring just over several generations. This points to environment as the major factor, and an environment that favors overeating and inactivity is fueling the worldwide diabetes epidemic.

So you can figure out when genetics are not on your side—if you have close relatives with diabetes, or if you are part of a high-risk ethnic group. And when you are at high risk and know it, developing a healthy lifestyle becomes all the more important. It has been said, "Genetics loads the gun, but environment pulls the trigger!" This is particularly true when it comes to diabetes. But there is a lot you can do to control your environment, and now we know for sure it works—the risk of diabetes can be effectively reduced.

Important new studies have shown scientifically how to prevent diabetes. Even when—maybe especially when—a person is well on his or her way to developing diabetes, progression to diabetes can be stopped in its tracks. And the good news is that it's not as hard as you may think. You don't have to go on a starvation diet or go into training for the Olympics to dramatically reduce your risk of developing type 2 diabetes.

The Proof That Diabetes Can Be Prevented

One sort of evidence comes from a large "observational study" at Harvard University. Researchers kept track of the lifestyle and health of more than 84,000 women for sixteen years, to see what factors predisposed them to diabetes. Women who maintained a healthy lifestyle as indicated by a healthy weight, good diet, regular physical activity, moderate alcohol use, and not smoking had 91-percent reduced risk of getting diabetes! Even those with a family history of diabetes had 88-percent reduced risk of diabetes if they lived a healthy lifestyle. This makes a very strong circumstantial case that type 2 diabetes can be prevented.

To really prove the point, though, randomized studies were needed that actually changed behavior of individual people. Over the past decade, there have been several of these, conducted throughout the world, among people with different nationalities and ethnic backgrounds. All support the notion that diabetes can be prevented. Here are some of the results:

■ In Malmo, Sweden, a healthy diet and increased physical activity reduced diabetes risk by more than half in 181 people with prediabetes over a six-year study period. These same interventions also restored normal glucose tolerance in 41 people with early-stage type 2 diabetes.

■ Among 577 people with prediabetes in Da Quing, China, a moderate program of diet only, exercise only, or a combination of diet plus exercise, reduced diabetes risk by 31 to 46 percent over a six-year period. People in the exercise-only and diet-plus-exercise groups fared better than people who made only dietary changes.

■ In Finland, 522 middle-aged, overweight men with prediabetes who adopted a healthy diet and a moderate exercise program, and who lost a modest amount of weight (about ten pounds), reduced their risk of developing diabetes by 58 percent over a 3.2-year study period.

THE DIABETES PREVENTION
PROGRAM (DPP)

The DPP holds a special place among studies showing that diabetes can be prevented. It is not only the largest such study yet conducted, but it compared both a lifestyle modification and a pharmacologic (drug) treatment. Maybe most important, the DPP included a broad cross-section of Americans—older, younger, Caucasian, African American, Latino, and Native American. This diversity of enrollment is important when you consider the different eating habits, food preferences, and physical activity levels of differing groups of Americans.

The DPP was also a model of well-designed, well-executed clinical research. DPP studied people who were screened because they had high-risk characteristics for diabetes. Everyone enrolled had impaired glucose tolerance on an oral glucose tolerance test; in other words if they had what we now call prediabetes. And once enrolled, participants were randomly assigned to one of four groups: *intensive lifestyle, metformin* (a pill that has been used for many years to treat diabetes, but not to prevent it), *troglitazone* (a new pill then being developed to treat diabetes), or *placebo pills.* After less than a year, troglitazone was stopped when unacceptable risk was discovered. The remaining three groups were followed closely for almost three years.

The intensive lifestyle group, with lots of dietary and exercise advice and encouragement, reduced their average daily intake by about 450 calories (the equivalent of a "large" order of fries or a cup of premium ice cream!), lost an average of about fifteen pounds, and maintained an average weight loss of ten pounds up to the end of the study. They also increased their activity level to the equivalent of walking about thirty minutes a day.

The drug-treated groups were also diligent in taking their pills, and the results were definitive: the group that had lost weight and exercised more had a 58-percent reduction in the rate of diabetes, while the group treated with metformin had a 31-percent reduction of diabetes.

The DPP proved once and for all that the risk of diabetes can be greatly reduced in high-risk people by moderate weight reduction and increased activity. Furthermore, diet and exercise was almost twice as effective at preventing diabetes than was taking the drug metformin. The study is continuing in a long-term follow-up phase to answer questions, such as whether this protective effect continues, and whether less heart disease can be found.

◼ In the Diabetes Prevention Program (DPP—see page 20) more than 3,000 overweight men and women with prediabetes reduced their daily calorie intake, exercised more, and maintained weight loss over a three-year period. As a result of these lifestyle modifications, the risk of progressing to diabetes was reduced by nearly 58 percent.

SMALL CHANGES CAN MAKE A BIG DIFFERENCE

All of the studies mentioned above emphasize that simple and modest lifestyle changes pay off with *big* dividends. Here is a summary of some of the specific lifestyle changes that have been encouraged in clinical trials to stop diabetes:

◼ Eat a healthy diet that is low in calories, fat, and saturated fat. Limit fat intake to 30 percent of calories and saturated fat to no more than 10 percent of calories. None of the studies tested specifically whether reducing fat or carbohydrate or both were most effective, but all emphasized limiting fat and total calories.

◼ Choose more vegetables, fruits, whole grains, lean meats, low-fat dairy products, and unsaturated fats.

◼ Increase fiber intake to 30 grams per day.

◼ Reduce intake of sugar.

◼ Engage in moderate-intensity physical activity, such as brisk walking, for at least 150 minutes each week (about 30 minutes 5 days a week).

IT'S NEVER TOO LATE TO STOP DIABETES

As people get older, their risk of developing type 2 diabetes rises dramatically. In fact, as many as one out of five people over age sixty have type 2 diabetes. Does this mean that older people benefit less from lifestyle change? Just the opposite. The DPP found that good nutrition and moderate exercise was even more effective in people age sixty and older than in younger people. The seniors lowered their risk of developing diabetes by more than 70 percent. In contrast, metformin was relatively ineffective in preventing diabetes in older people and more effective in the younger and more overweight people.

■ Lose at least 5 percent of body weight (the equivalent of a 10-pound weight loss for a 200-pound person).

Although these strategies seem simple and straightforward, anyone who has tried to implement them on a permanent basis knows they can be easier said than done. This is why study participants met regularly with "lifestyle coaches," (who were usually registered dietitians) and other health-care professionals who could help them set goals and devise strategies tailored to their individual needs and lifestyle. They had access to group courses and individualized instruction on healthy eating, exercise, weight loss, stress management, behavior change, and relapse prevention. Most important, lifestyle change was viewed as an ongoing, long-term proposition rather than a quick fix.

Does More Effort Mean More Benefit?

What happens if you choose to make more dramatic lifestyle modifications than those advocated in clinical trials to stop diabetes? What if you lose more than 5 percent of your body weight, exercise an hour a day, and more closely adhere to a healthy diet? Could you reduce your risk of diabetes even more? Very likely. In fact, in the Finnish Diabetes Prevention Study, the more successful the study participants were at achieving their lifestyle goals, the better they were able to prevent diabetes from developing. For instance, people who lost more than 5 percent of their initial weight were 70 percent less likely to develop diabetes than people who lost little or no weight, and people who were the most physically active (more than four hours per week) cut their risk of diabetes by 80 percent—even if they did not lose weight.

Good sense suggests, though, that the added effect of very rigorous lifestyle changes will only last if the healthy lifestyle is maintained. Crash diets or exercise programs followed by periods of weight gain and apathy, one could reasonably assume, do not work. So the sustainability of a lifestyle change has to be considered.

Improving Your Health Outlook in a Matter of Weeks with Lifestyle Changes

Motivated people who start making lifestyle changes can reap tremendous health benefits almost immediately. In one study, people who ate a low-fat, high-fiber diet and added forty-five to sixty minutes of physical activity to their day were able to significantly reduce their blood pressure, improve their cholesterol levels, and lower their blood insulin levels in just three weeks. In fact it's been proven over and over again that a low-calorie diet and increased physical activity lowers blood glucose levels within weeks, even before significant weight loss. To see the continued benefit, you do want to keep the weight curve on the downslope.

Drugs Versus Diet and Lifestyle Changes

The search is underway for drugs that can halt the progression to diabetes, and there are some promising candidates. But so far, drug therapy has proven to be less effective than lifestyle modification. In addition, drug therapy always carries the risk of side effects. And of course there's the expense of purchasing medications, which can be considerable. At this point, the FDA has not approved any pills for the indication of preventing diabetes, so it is not likely that insurers will pay for them unless they already have diabetes.

Here are some of the diabetes-fighting drugs that have been tested so far.

- *Metformin.* Metformin is a diabetes drug that improves insulin action, especially on the liver. The DPP showed that people who took metformin reduced their risk of progressing to diabetes by 31 percent (although the program of positive lifestyle change was nearly twice as effective as the drug therapy). Metformin was most effective in younger, heavier people and less effective in older, less overweight people. Metformin often causes loose stools or diarrhea and cannot be taken by people with kidney disease or in several other situations, because of the potential to cause a rare but serious problem known as lactic acidosis.
- *Acarbose.* This drug slows the absorption of carbohydrate from foods, resulting in lower blood sugar levels after meals. In clinical studies, people who take

acarbose three times a day were 25 to 32 percent less likely to develop diabetes than people who take a placebo. Acarbose also helps some people who have IGT revert back to normal glucose tolerance. Side effects of the drug, however, include gastrointestinal problems like flatulence and diarrhea.

■ *Troglitazone.* The DPP and other studies showed that this drug, which makes cells more responsive to insulin, can reduce the progression to diabetes by more than 50 percent. However, troglitazone has been removed from the market because of a potential to cause severe liver damage. There are other drugs in this class, such as rosiglitazone and pioglitazone, but their effect on preventing diabetes is yet to be shown.

It should be understood, when you consider drug therapy, that the moderate positive lifestyle changes we consider the best approach cost nothing extra, have no adverse side effects (unless an occasional stiff muscle is called an adverse effect), and help prevent heart disease, cancer, and many other health problems—making lifestyle change the clear winner in the fight against diabetes.

Can Diabetes Be Prevented Indefinitely?

No one knows yet. So far, clinical trials have proven that diabetes can be delayed, for at least six years, and longer-term follow-up will give more insight into this important question. But any delay in the occurrence of diabetes should help in staving off complications like cardiovascular disease, kidney disease, blindness, and nerve damage. And in some people, a healthy lifestyle may prevent diabetes permanently. We just don't know for sure yet.

Getting the Help You Need

Long-term change can be difficult. This is why it's smart to seek help when you need it. Your physician can be a primary resource and support person, discussing your risk for diabetes and screening with a fasting plasma glucose or even an oral glucose tolerance test (see chapter 1). A registered dietitian or licensed nutritionist is best at working with you on exactly what changes are most promising in your own case. Because everyone is different, every meal plan is different. You may be very surprised to learn what you *can* have in your own meal plan, as well as where the bulk of your own caloric intake is coming from. Other professionals, whether exercise specialists, podiatrists, mental health counselors or others, may also help you meet your goals. As always, if you don't feel you are getting what you need in professional help, or if you doubt their qualifications or professionalism, shop around. There is plenty of good, professional help out there.

How much and what type of help you need will depend on your own personal situation. Managed-care organizations or health-insurance providers often offer access to a variety of health-care professionals at little or no charge. They may also have arrangements with local health clubs and weight-loss programs to help you obtain discounts for memberships and services. Remember that it's up to you to search out the help you need and up to you, in the end, to decide to make the changes.

The Bottom Line: Recommendations for Preventing Diabetes

Studies have proven unequivocally that type 2 diabetes can be prevented or at least delayed for years. Even small changes in lifestyle can produce big results. Preventing diabetes boils down to a trio of simple strategies, listed below. These strategies can be phased in at your own pace and need not be overwhelming. The remaining chapters in this book will help you find simple ways to implement these changes in your everyday life.

1. **Keep Your Weight in Check.** Obesity, and the resulting insulin resistance, is the underlying cause of most cases of diabetes. Losing weight helps reduce insulin resistance, so cells can remove glucose from the blood more efficiently. Even a ten- to fifteen-pound weight loss can make a dramatic difference in your diabetes risk. Chapter 6 will help you determine what a healthy body weight is and will provide plenty of tips for helping you get there. We will give you many of the secrets of losing weight and keeping it off. In fact, here are the two most important, if not secret, approaches:

2. **Be Physically Active.** Physical activity combats insulin resistance, so cells can remove glucose from the blood more efficiently. Even if you don't lose weight, regular exercise can substantially reduce your risk for diabetes. Chapter 4 will guide

you in getting the activity you need to ward off diabetes. As you will see, exercise does not have to be an ordeal, consume a lot of time, or cost a lot of money.

3. **Eat Smart.** *What* and *how much* you eat can both affect diabetes risk, but adopting a prudent eating plan need not mean dieting and deprivation. Furthermore, some general rules apply to eating for diabetes prevention, but one diet does not fit all. Chapter 4 will help you separate fact from fiction when it comes to fighting diabetes with food.

Studies conducted among diverse populations throughout the world absolutely demonstrate that type 2 diabetes can be prevented. Best of all, you don't have to spend hours in a gym or go on an extreme diet to stop diabetes in its tracks. As the following chapters will show, making a few simple changes can provide a huge return on your investment.

3. TIPPING THE SCALES IN YOUR FAVOR

Obesity now rivals—and will soon surpass—smoking as the number-one cause of preventable death among Americans. One reason is the dramatic rise in diabetes risk that accompanies weight gain. The good news is that losing even a small amount of weight can substantially reduce your chances of developing diabetes.

Your Weight—How Much Is Too Much?

The relationship between excess body weight and diabetes is dramatic—it shows up in research any way you look at the problem. The more overweight, the greater the risk. For a single individual, gaining weight increases the chance of diabetes. For a whole nation, the heavier the average person, the more diabetes shows up (diabetes is unusual in undernourished parts of the world, and most common in the so-called developed world). People who emigrate from their native land to America, such as Japanese Americans, have also been studied, and the result is the same: the more weight they gain on the Western diet, the more diabetes.

How does being overweight raise diabetes risk? As the body accumulates excess fat, cells become increasingly resistant to the effects of insulin (insulin resistance). As we emphasized in Chapter 1, this means the pancreas must work harder to secrete enough extra insulin to remove sugar from the blood. Over time, the pancreas can no longer keep up with this increased insulin demand, so blood sugar levels rise and diabetes results.

How do you know what a healthy body weight is for you? One of the simplest methods used by health professionals is determining the body mass index (BMI). BMI is an expression of body weight relative to height. For most people, the higher the BMI, the more body fat they carry. You can use a simple formula to determine your body mass index:

BMI = [Weight in pounds ÷ Height in inches ÷ Height in inches] × 703

You can do this calculation in three easy steps:

1. Divide your weight (in pounds) by your height (in inches)
2. Divide the resulting number by your height in inches once again.
3. Multiply the resulting number by 703 to get your BMI.

For a person who is 5 feet 6 inches (66 inches) tall and weighs 160 pounds the calculation would be:

160 divided by 66 = 2.42, then 2.42 divided by 66 = 0.0366, then 0.0366 x 703 = 25.8

Many Internet sites, such as the Centers for Disease Control, provide more information on the BMI and feature online BMI calculators (*http://www.cdc.gov/nccdphp/dnpa/bmi/ index.htm*). Page 234 also presents a BMI chart, which you can use to quickly look up a range of BMIs.

So now you know your BMI. What does it mean? BMIs between 19 and 25 are associated with the longest, healthiest life spans. A BMI of 25 to 29.9 places you in the overweight category and greatly raises your risk of developing diabetes, high blood pressure, heart disease, and other health problems. A BMI of 30 or more indicates an even more serious classification of obesity.

Limitations of the BMI

The BMI correlates well with percentage of body fat but it should not be interpreted as a precise measure of body fat. The reason? Age, gender, and level of physical fitness affect the relation between body fatness and BMI. For instance, women usually have a higher percent of body fat than men for the same BMI. Older people usually have more body fat than younger adults, and sedentary people will have more body fat than fit people like athletes and weight lifters. Nonetheless, the BMI is a good screening tool and indicator of risk for obesity-related health problems for the general population.

Another limitation to the BMI is that it doesn't consider *where* on the body the fat is stored. People who store fat around their middle (the so-called "apple" shape) are at an especially high risk for diabetes and cardiovascular disease. Those with the fat in their hips and thighs ("pear" shape) are at less risk. In fact, some studies show that waist circumference is a stronger predictor of diabetes risk than is body mass index. Men who

BMI CLASSIFICATIONS		
CLASSIFICATION	BMI RANGE	COMMENTS
Healthy weight	18.5–24.9	Maintain your weight within this range if possible. People who have a BMI between 18.5 and 21.9 are at the very lowest risk for developing diabetes.
Overweight	25–29.9	In this BMI range, diabetes risk more than triples compared to the healthy weight range. Avoid any additional weight gain and try to gradually reduce your weight.
Obese	≥30	When BMI reaches 30 to 34.9 diabetes risk increases up to twentyfold. At a BMI of 35 or higher, risk can rise fortyfold. Start working on a program of gradual weight loss.

have a waist circumference of 40 inches or more and women who have a waist of 35 inches or more are at an especially high risk.

For the most precise measure of body fat, you can have your percentage of body fat tested. A health professional such as a registered dietitian or exercise physiologist can sometimes do this for you. The body fat percentages associated with the lowest health risks are between 12 and 20 percent for men and 20 to 30 percent for women, with the lower ends of these ranges being the most desirable.

BMI and Children

The BMI calculation presented above for adults does not work with children because the interpretation of BMI depends on the child's age. Boys and girls also differ in degree of body fat as they grow and mature. For these reasons, BMIs for children must be plotted on gender-specific growth charts. A health-care professional can assist you in assessing your child's BMI and weight status.

Is There Such a Thing as Too Much Weight Loss?

Definitely! Throughout this book, we emphasize the benefits of weight control, but our basic assumption is that we are talking to people who are overweight. Anorexia nervosa is the psychiatric diagnosis for people who are obsessed with losing weight *even though they are already normal or underweight.* Make no mistake: Anorexia nervosa is a serious, potentially fatal illness that requires intensive psychiatric care. So be on the lookout for its signs in people you know or even in yourself. Striving to achieve *normal* body weight is one thing, a good thing. But striving to lose even more weight when you are normal or underweight can be very, very dangerous.

The Final Word on Your Healthy Weight

Before making any final decision about your ideal body weight, consult your physician or dietitian. If you have been overweight for many years, a realistic body weight might be somewhat higher than the BMI recommendations presented above. But realize that if you lose just 5 to 10 percent of your body weight and keep it off, you can reap significant health benefits.

Weight Loss—What Works?

We are a nation obsessed with weight. A recent survey reported that 78 percent of women and 64 percent of men are currently trying to lose or maintain their weight. Well over 30 billion dollars are spent each year on weight-loss products and services. Why, then, are so few people successful at losing weight and keeping it off? This section will take a look at why diets often fail and discuss the pros and cons of some popular weight-loss diet strategies.

Most people who struggle with their weight have tried numerous diets and lost significant amounts of weight at one time or another. Low-fat, low-carb, high-protein, meal replacement shakes, and even a diet of cabbage soup or Subway sandwiches can all produce results. *All diets work because they limit something and people end up eating fewer calories than they expend.* Unfortunately, these limitations are the very reason that most people cannot maintain a diet long term. Still, many of these diets contain pearls of wisdom that can be applied to a program that produces long-term results. Let's look at some popular weight-loss strategies, highlight the most useful parts of each one, and put them together into a plan that makes sense.

LOW-FAT DIETS

The premise of these diets is that fat is a concentrated source of calories (9 calories per gram compared with 4 for carbohydrate and protein), so cutting back on high-fat foods will usually cut caloric intake and promote weight loss. The problem is in the "usually"— if you are not careful, it's easy to go overboard with extra carbs—fat-free and low-fat bread, snack foods, and sweets. Many of these foods are loaded with sugar and white flour and contain just as many calories as the higher-fat versions. In addition, these carbohydrate foods cause a rapid rise in blood sugar and insulin levels that can actually trigger hunger and lead to a roller-coaster pattern of overeating. This is why some people feel like they are "addicted" to carbohydrates. Adding insult to injury, refined carbs can contribute to numerous other health problems, such as high triglycerides and low HDL (good) cholesterol. Many people also find a very low-fat diet difficult to follow without feeling deprived, making it tough to stick with it long-term.

On the other hand, many low-fat foods are excellent choices for a weight-loss program, and the best long-term results in preventing diabetes, the Diabetes Prevention Program, concentrates on reducing fat calories *without* increasing the carbohydrates. Vegetables, fruits, whole grains, lean-protein foods, and low-fat dairy products should be staples in a healthy, low-fat diet. A diet that emphasizes these foods plus those with small to moderate amounts of "good" fats such as nuts and seeds and healthful vegetable oils will be high in fiber and disease-fighting nutrients, low in calories, and much easier to live with long-term. The bottom line is that done right, a low-fat diet can promote weight loss—done wrong, it can be a disaster.

LOW-CARB DIETS

These diets advocate reducing carbohydrate intake to lower blood insulin levels and promote the breakdown of stored fat. Refined carbohydrates like sugar and white flour are especially banned. The most extreme form of this regimen allows dieters to eat unlimited amounts of high-fat meat, cheese, cream, butter, and eggs, but only very small portions of vegetables—and no fruit, grain products, or milk at all.

On the plus side, this diet promotes rapid weight loss. During the first week, much of the lost weight is water, but after that, a significant amount of fat is lost too— *if* the total calories are reduced. Because the diet is so high in protein, it is very filling and most people are not physically hungry. In addition, after a few days of severe carbohydrate restriction, people go into a state of ketosis, a state in which the body burns fat as its primary fuel. The ketones (the chemicals produced when the body is in ketosis) that begin to circulate in the blood also have an appetite-suppressant effect. The net effect is that most people end up eating fewer calories than they normally do. Some studies also show that low-carb, high-protein diets help prevent the drop in metabolic rate seen with high-carb weight-loss diets. Higher-protein diets also appear to preserve lean body mass better.

But there are many downsides to an extremely low-carb high-protein diet, some of which are at this point just theoretical while others are very real and practical:

■ If you have diabetes and take insulin or oral medications, blood sugar levels drop very rapidly, so you would have to work with your health-care provider to adjust doses.

■ Because of rapid water loss from the body, high blood pressure medications may need adjusting under a physician's supervision.

- The low-fiber content of the diet makes constipation a pervasive problem.
- Rapid water loss can lead to dehydration.
- Electrolyte imbalances, partly due to rapid water loss, can cause leg cramps and other problems.
- The high-protein content and diuretic effect of the diet can precipitate an attack of gout.
- As muscle carbohydrate stores become depleted, weakness and low energy often result, making it difficult to exercise.
- Eating excessive amounts of protein can burden the kidneys and liver.
- The diet is very low in fiber, vitamins, minerals, antioxidants, and phyto-chemicals, so requires nutritional supplementation.
- A diet high in fatty meats, butter, and cream is high in saturated fat and may be associated with a higher risk of cardiovascular disease, colon cancer, and Alzheimer's disease.
- Some research suggests that high-fat meals can cause arteries to stiffen for several hours after eating. When arteries lose their ability to expand and con-tract, the workload of the heart increases, possibly even raising the risk for heart attack.
- Eating high on the food chain increases your exposure to environmental tox-ins, which are especially concentrated in the fatty portion of meats and dairy products.

Probably most significant for the long-term effect of the very low-carbohydrate diet is that it is *very* restricted, and most people end up "cheating" before long, making this just another fad-diet phase. However, the basic principle of this diet is definitely worth sav-ing: fats are not toxic; you can reduce carbohydrates and do well. Do include some pro-tein in meals and snacks. This will help suppress your appetite, keep your metabolic rate from dropping, and preserve muscle mass. But instead of a low-carb, high-fat free-for-all, opt for skinless poultry; fish; lean beef and pork; and low-fat milk, yogurt, and cheese. Balance the protein out with moderate amounts of "good" carbs (vegetables, fruits, legumes, and whole grains) and healthy fats, and you are much more likely to have a plan for long-term success.

MEAL-REPLACEMENT DIETS

Many people enjoy the ease of using diet shakes and bars to replace one or two meals a day. Variations of this diet include substituting foods like frozen low-calorie meals or a fixed sandwich or cereal for a couple of meals every day. Replacing meals with shakes or specific foods eliminates the stress of meal planning and helps people keep calories under control.

A main advantage to meal replacement diets is that they are fixed—in content, in calories, and in amount. They help some people regain control over eating. And contrary to popular belief, variety is not always the spice of life. In fact, studies show that the greater variety of foods a person is exposed to, the more likely they will be to overeat. This is why buffets and food bars are such a disaster for dieters.

A disadvantage to over-reliance on meal replacements or rigid menus with no variety is that it could lead to nutritional deficiencies—or even excess—over time. Some of the bars and shakes that are available today are high in artificial ingredients and sugar and are more like glorified candy bars or milkshakes than meals. Other products contain excessive amounts of added vitamins, minerals, and herbal ingredients that could actually be harmful if eaten too often. A potential pitfall of eating the same food every day is exposure to unknown harmful constituents. For instance, a person who eats a certain kind of fish every day might unknowingly expose themselves to high levels of mercury or other environmental contaminants.

The take-home message from this diet is that relying on a very fixed, very repetitive meal for part of your total nutrition intake may help you gain better control of your overall eating habits. Having just one or two standard, carefully selected breakfasts, lunches, and dinners that you enjoy for your basic diet can be helpful. However, it's smart to rotate in new foods periodically to assure dietary balance and limit exposure to unknown harmful substances. If you want to use meal replacement shakes or bars, check with your dietitian to see how these products can safely fit into your eating plan.

Strategies for Weight-Loss Success

Any diet can produce weight loss in the short term. But to ensure continued success and *permanent* weight loss, you must find an eating plan you can adopt for life, and it must limit the calories. This section will help you do just that by outlining the most effective strategies for long-term success.

VEGETABLES AND FRUITS—WHAT'S A SERVING?

Five a day is the minimum recommended amount. But to optimize your health, aim for seven to ten servings. This is not as hard as you may think; each of the following constitutes a serving:

- 1 cup leafy salad greens
- ½ cup cooked or raw fruits or vegetables
- ½ cup cooked dried beans or peas
- 1 medium piece of fruit such as apple, peach, or orange
- ¼ cup dried fruit
- ¾ cup fruit or vegetable juice

Using the above guidelines, a large chef salad made with 3 cups of lettuce plus a cup of other chopped vegetables like mushrooms, onions, carrots, and tomatoes, equals five servings. A meal that contains a cup of steamed broccoli plus a medium baked sweet potato equals 4 servings. If you include at least one cup of vegetables or fruit at each meal and replace snacks like pretzels, crackers, chips, and cookies with fruits and vegetables, you will easily meet or exceed the daily recommendation.

PILE ON THE PRODUCE

Eating plenty of produce is one of your best weapons against the battle of the bulge. Low in calories and high in bulk, these foods will fill you up but not out. People who skip the vegetables and fruits at a mere 25 to 50 calories per cup and pile on extra rice or pasta at 200 calories per cup—or who have an extra slice of bread at 80 to 100 calories—will probably find weight loss slower than they expect. Realize that starchy vegetables like potatoes, corn, and peas contain about the same amount of calories and carbs as rice or pasta, so think of these foods as bread, rice, or pasta substitutes. Reserve half your plate at each meal for vegetables and fruits and aim for seven to ten servings a day.

PACK SOME PROTEIN INTO MEALS AND SNACKS

Protein-rich foods are the most filling of all foods, so they stave off hunger and keep you feeling satisfied until your next meal. Replacing some of the carbohydrate in meals and snacks with protein will also keep your metabolism revved up and help you maintain muscle while losing fat. There's no need to go overboard and completely eliminate carbs, though. Just choose appropriate portions of healthy "good carbs," which are high in fiber and low in calories. The menus in the Sample Menus section will help you plan protein-packed meals to meet your weight-loss goals.

To keep calories under control, be sure to choose skinless poultry; lean cuts of beef and pork; fish and seafood; egg whites and fat-free egg substitutes; and low-fat milk, cheese, and yogurt. To get a healthy balance of nutrients, substitute vegetarian alternatives like legumes, tofu, and veggie burgers for meat frequently.

GO FOR THE *WHOLE* GRAIN

People who eat whole grains instead of refined versions have less insulin resistance, and lower diabetes risk, and tend to be thinner. Why? Whole grains—like brown rice, oatmeal, and whole wheat—provide far more fiber and nutrients than their refined counterparts. The fiber in whole grains also provides a feeling of fullness that sustains you between meals. On the other hand, a diet of refined low-fiber foods like white bread, refined breakfast cereal, and toaster pastries can actually stimulate hunger by causing wide swings in blood sugar levels.

Chapter 5 will guide you in choosing the best whole-grain products in your grocery store. The recipes and menus in this book provide many delicious ways to enjoy the goodness of whole grains.

SERVE UP SOME CALCIUM

While its claim to fame is building strong bones, calcium can also help reduce high blood pressure and may protect against insulin resistance. New research also suggests that high-calcium diets may fight obesity by encouraging cells to burn fat rather than store it. One study found that each 300-milligram increase in daily calcium intake (the equivalent of one cup of milk) was associated with about two pounds less body fat in children and five to six pounds less body fat in adults.

What's the best way to get your calcium? The fat-fighting effects of calcium appear to be greatest when consumed in foods rather than in supplements. Dairy products such as *low-fat* milk, yogurt, and cheese are an excellent source—aim for two to three servings per day. Other calcium-rich foods include greens, calcium-fortified soy foods, and legumes. If necessary, take enough supplemental calcium to bring your intake up to the recommended daily amount. Adults up to age fifty should aim for 1,000 milligrams per day. After age fifty, the calcium requirement increases to 1,200 milligrams per day.

Begin Your Day with Breakfast

Many people who are trying to lose weight skip breakfast thinking this is a good way to cut calories. But this strategy can backfire in a big way. The key to dieting is your total number of calories in a day, and if skipping breakfast just sets you up to feel hungry and overeat at lunch or supper, then the result is more negative than positive. Rather than skip breakfast, choose a better breakfast—featuring fiber-rich foods, lean proteins, and limited calories. Chapter 8 and the Sample Menus section present plenty of recipes and menu ideas that will keep you feeling full and satisfied all morning long.

Snack Smart

One of the best secrets of successful weight loss is to substitute healthful snacks like fruits, yogurt, vegetables, and low-fat popcorn for refined carbohydrate snacks like sweets, sodas, chips, pretzels, and crackers. Why? Replacing high-fat, high-carb snack foods with "good carbs" will help stabilize blood sugar and insulin levels and help prevent hunger. The appendix presents sample menus with smart snack suggestions.

The timing of snacks is also important. Especially avoid late-night snacking. Make it a policy to stop eating at least three hours before bedtime. Overeating in the evening is the main reason that many people aren't hungry for breakfast in the morning. This habit creates an eating pattern where the majority of calories are consumed later in the day, a major impediment to weight-loss success.

Trim the Fat

Trimming unnecessary fat is a key strategy for keeping calories under control. How important is cutting back on fat? With 9 calories per gram, fat has more than twice the calories of carbohydrate or protein, which is why foods like oil, butter, and mayonnaise can pack a lot of calories into a very small portion.

Researchers have discovered that people who successfully lose weight and keep it off *do* watch their fat intake. In fact, weight-loss maintainers limit their fat intake to about 25 percent of calories. See chapter 3 for more on which fats are best and which to avoid.

When trimming your fat intake, beware of the "fat-free" trap. Realize that just because a food is low in fat does not mean it is good for you. Many fat-free foods like pretzels, crackers, breads, cookies, sodas, and candies are naturally without fat, just as lard is without carbohydrate. These "fat-free" foods may be excessively high in carbohydrates and sugar. They may not be filling and can actually trigger hunger.

Avoid Portion Distortion

Food portions have grown dramatically over the past several decades (see the table below). Even appliances and bakeware are bigger today. For instance, toasters now have extra wide slots to accommodate supersize bagels and extra-thick bread slices. Muffin, cake, and pie pans are made in larger sizes, too. Dinner plates, mugs, and glasses have also grown in size. All this means there's probably more food on your plate than there was a couple of decades ago. Fight back by using smaller plates and serving up smaller portions. When eating out, split a meal with a friend.

PORTION PROBLEMS		
Food	1950s	Now
Fast-food burger patty	Less than 2 ounces	6 to 8 ounces
Soda	8 ounces	32 to 64 ounces
Movie popcorn	3 cups	16 cups
Muffin	Less than 1½ ounces	5 to 8 ounces

SERVING SAVVY

Studies show that if it's on your plate, you will most likely eat it. In fact, people eat about 30 percent more food when they start out with a large plate of food instead of beginning with only a small portion. This is why it's best to start out with a conservative portion. You can always have a little more if you are still truly hungry, but if you start out with a big portion, you will probably clean your plate, even if you aren't all that hungry.

WATER—DON'T LEAVE HOME WITHOUT IT

Many people eat when they're really just thirsty. Drinking enough fluids will help prevent this kind of overeating and has some side benefits also. It fills the stomach, at least for a while; and it gives you something to ingest that isn't necessarily caloric. What should you drink? Water (plain or with a wedge of lemon or lime) is the best choice since it is calorie-free. Unsweetened tea is another good choice. Most people can consume caffeinated beverages in moderation without harm, but check with your physicain or dietitian if you have any doubts.

How much fluid is enough? For most people, six to eight cups daily is sufficient. If your urine is a pale yellow color (like lemonade) this is a sign that you are well hydrated.

A SIMPLE DIFFERENCE: DIET OR NONDIET DRINKS?

It is remarkable how many people do not quite get the simple difference between diet and nondiet drinks. We often see people who are quenching the thirst of uncontrolled diabetes with regular soda or orange juice—not a good choice, because they are almost pure sugar. Diet sodas, on the other hand, provide 0 calories or sugar. So just check out the label . . . if it says 0 calories, that's the answer. Of course water is the surest no-cal drink!

Avoid beverages that contain calories—like sugary sodas, juice drinks, and fruit juices—because these are not filling or satisfying compared to solid foods, making it easy to over-consume calories.

Slow Down to Fill Up

"Behavior modification" is a psychological treatment that works, and it does not take a whole lot of counseling. It involves techniques like just eating more slowly than you are used to. Chew your food thoroughly, put down your fork or spoon between bites. Sound easy? Well, it's not easy to change the actual physical way you eat, but it is remarkably effective. It takes about twenty minutes for the stomach to signal the brain that you're full, and in the meantime if you've been eating at a fast and furious rate, you quickly become overstuffed. In limiting how much you eat, you may enjoy some conversation along the way. It is a fact that people who eat too quickly consume more food than they need and feel uncomfortably full afterward. So try some behavior modification on yourself. Eat at half the rate you usually do. Put down your fork between every bite. Enjoy some conversation or a good read. It will definitely help.

Be Cognizant of Calories

Most people don't gain weight overnight—it usually creeps up by a couple of pounds a year. And it's not hard to do. Eating just 100 extra calories per day beyond what you will need can result in a ten-pound weight gain over the course of a year! Perhaps the most painless way to start shedding pounds is to find a way to trim 100 calories from your daily diet *or* burn 100 calories more with physical activity. Even better, do both. Cutting back a little on portions, substituting healthful lower-calorie foods for high-calorie versions, or walking more throughout the day easily accomplishes this. The table on page 41 shows the impact of making specific changes on a daily basis over the course of a year. (It assumes that you don't make up extra calories in some other way, of course.) But as you can see, small changes can make a *big* difference.

Get Moving

There's no getting around it. Physical activity is a must for weight-loss success. Besides burning calories, exercise promotes a healthy body weight by building muscle mass

INSTEAD OF . . .	SUBSTITUTE . . .	POUNDS LOST PER YEAR
Sausage & Egg Biscuit	Egg sandwich on a whole wheat English muffin	20
Medium cheeseburger & fries	Low-fat turkey & cheese sandwich with a cup of vegetable soup	38
12-oz sugared soda	Water	14
1 cup superpremium ice cream	1 cup low-fat ice cream	34
1 ounce potato chips	3 cups low-fat popcorn	8
4 low-fat cookies	Medium apple	12
1 tablespoon regular mayonnaise	1 tablespoon nonfat mayonnaise	9
Watching television	30-minute walk	12
Sitting at computer	30 minutes playing basketball	24

(which raises your metabolic rate) and by helping to reduce stress, which is a major cause of overeating. How much exercise is enough? Thirty minutes a day is the minimum recommended amount, but people who successfully lose weight and keep it off often do about twice this much. Chapter 7 provides more information about working exercise into your life.

Losing Weight—Beyond Diet and Exercise

"Diet" and "exercise" are the first things that usually come to mind when people think of losing weight. However, a couple of other factors are absolutely fundamental and lay the groundwork for weight-loss success. Paying attention to these two very important issues can mean the difference between success and failure.

STRESS AND YOUR WEIGHT

It's no secret that stress is a major cause of overeating. And it's not tuna fish and salad that stressed-out people crave—it's cookies, ice cream, and chips. Research may someday unravel why stress sends many people seeking sugary, fatty foods; but if you need reminding, just try spelling *stressed* backward. You got it . . . *desserts*!

Stress does cause the body to release various hormones that enable the body to cope—the "fight-or-flight response." One of these hormones, *cortisol,* triggers appetite and favors fat storage around the belly. Some experts believe that cortisol may be involved in the adverse effects of stress, the added pounds around your midsection, the development of metabolic syndrome, cardiovascular disease, and even diabetes. But whether stress causes specific hormone responses that promote weight gain, or just bad decision-making in what you eat, there is no doubt that stress interferes with weight control.

Even obsessing about diet and weight loss can stress you out making your weight-loss efforts much more difficult. This is why it's so important to have a relaxed attitude, focus on eating well for good health, be patient, and be content with slow but steady weight loss. Find ways to simplify your life, learn to relax, and deal with emotional issues so they don't block your weight-loss program. This may be as important as nutrition and exercise in the long run.

HOW SLEEP DEPRIVATION CAN PUT ON POUNDS

For some people, the key to better weight control might just lie in a good night's sleep. Why? People who feel fatigued all day often snack in an effort to gain energy and increase alertness. There are a series of hormonal reactions to lack of sleep that could play a role: increased cortisol, lower growth hormone, for example. Finally, and maybe most important of all, people with insomnia are often in the habit of getting up for the traditional "midnight snack," which can easily add 500 calories to a day's intake. Remember, with 500 extra calories, it only takes a week to gain a pound, and in three months you're twelve pounds heavier.

The bottom line is sleep deprivation can put on pounds. You can eat well and exercise with the best of intentions, but if you don't get enough rest, you won't get the maximum benefit from your weight-loss attempts.

What If You Can't Lose Weight?

Despite good intentions and valiant attempts, many people have a *very* difficult time losing weight. If this is your experience, it may be time to try a different approach. Instead of trying to lose weight, try to halt any upward creep and focus on maintaining your current weight. The combination of a good diet and regular physical activity can substantially reduce your diabetes risk even if you remain overweight. You may even find that removing the pressure to lose weight while moving toward a better quality diet and more active lifestyle could stimulate weight loss without really even trying.

People who are struggling with their weight can also consult with a registered dietitian who specializes in weight management. She or he can evaluate your diet, set realistic goals, and help you devise a personalized plan for success. Remember that losing as little as ten to fifteen pounds in combination with a healthy diet and regular moderate exercise can reduce diabetes risk by nearly 60 percent.

"THERE'S SOMETHING IN ME THAT WANTS TO GAIN BACK THE WEIGHT!"

Unfortunately, medical studies are finding that it's true: The body has a natural tendency to gain back weight lost through vigorous dieting. There are new hormones, with odd names like "leptin," "adeponectin," and "grehlin," that help explain this "homing instinct" of the body to regain weight. Someday, the research may lead to effective weight-controlling drugs. But in the meantime, it's worth understanding that the kind of diet and the kind of activity we suggest throughout this book—high in vegetables, fruits, and whole grains, and lots of moving around—are really the *natural* human condition. It is *unnatural* to sit around all day and eat refined, fatty foods. You should also be heartened to know that many, many people have successfully changed their dietary and lifestyle patterns in healthier directions, successfully losing weight and keeping it off.

WEIGHT-LOSS CASE STUDY

Jan, a forty-year-old office manager, decided it was time to make some lifestyle changes. Her mother and older sister both suffered from type 2 diabetes, and while Jan's blood sugar was still within the normal range, she was eager to head things off at the pass. During her last physical, Jan discovered that she had elevated triglycerides and low HDL (good) cholesterol. Her doctor warned her that this could mean she was on her way to developing heart disease and diabetes. Jan's weight had also crept up after the births of her two children and she wanted to lose about twenty-five pounds.

Jan consulted a registered dietitian, who helped her take a good look at her eating patterns and lifestyle habits. Jan "craved carbohydrates" and tended to graze on foods like bagels, cereal bars, crackers, and pretzels. She avoided eating protein foods because she thought they were "fattening." In an effort to lose weight, she also skipped breakfast most days, but by lunch she felt very hungry, so she would usually treat herself to French fries along with her usual fast-food cheeseburger. In the afternoon, a snack would stave off feelings of overwhelming fatigue and sleepiness.

Jan's dietitian emphasized that her current diet was heavy in refined carbohydrates and quite high in fat. Overall, Jan was consuming some 2,500 calories, although if you had asked her she would have estimated 1,500. Furthermore, the pattern of eating was actually contributing to her cravings. Jan's dietitian pointed out that skipping breakfast made matters worse by causing the excess hunger at lunch. Though skeptical, Jan agreed to start eating breakfast. She also restructured her eating plan to include some protein in meals and small, healthy snacks. She replaced most of the starchy refined carbohydrates with vegetables, fruits, and whole grains.

From the very first day, Jan noticed a difference. Her low-fat breakfast omelette and bowl of fruit kept her full until lunchtime. A grilled chicken salad at lunch eliminated the need for a pack of vending machine crackers and soda later in the day. A late afternoon snack of low-fat cheese and whole grain crackers prevented overeating at dinner.

Jan also looked for ways to increase her activity level. At work she took the stairs instead of the elevator. She walked with a coworker during morning and afternoon breaks. She started walking the dog for thirty minutes most evenings after work and took up tennis after a ten-year hiatus. Over the next four months, Jan lost the excess weight and her blood lipids returned to normal. She was amazed that she no longer craved carbohydrates and she felt more energized than she had in years.

Secrets of Successful Losers

Most people can lose weight, but few can keep it off long-term. Why is it so hard to maintain weight loss? Researchers are looking at the reasons and scrutinizing the habits of "successful losers."

The best source of weight-loss secrets comes from the National Weight Control Registry (NWCR). The average NWCR participant has lost over 60 pounds and maintained their weight loss for over five years. How do they keep the weight off? So far, researchers have identified four habits that successful losers have in common:

- They watch their fat intake. On average, successful losers get about 25 percent of their calories from fat. They avoid fried foods, choose lean meats and low-fat dairy products, and replace other fatty foods with lighter versions.
- They eat breakfast, which helps them avoid overeating later in the day.
- They exercise for an hour a day. Successful weight-loss maintainers burn about 2,700 calories a week in physical activity, the equivalent of about a four-mile walk daily.
- They monitor their weight frequently and keep track of what they are eating. This allows them to catch problems early and do something about it.

Weight loss was accomplished by a variety of means—some people sought professional help and some did it on their own. They used various strategies including limiting foods high in fat and sugar, counting calories, and watching portions. Nearly everyone increased his or her activity level to help shed pounds. Incidentally, most NWCR participants had numerous unsuccessful attempts at losing weight before finally getting it right.

Do successful losers find weight maintenance a chore? Most find that the longer they keep their weight off the easier it becomes, as their new habits become more firmly ingrained.

Putting It All Together

We repeatedly emphasize that being overweight is the single biggest risk factor for type 2 diabetes. However, losing as little as ten pounds and keeping it off can significantly reduce your risk. No one knows the *best* way to lose weight, the best diet, and it is very likely that different approaches work for different people. Experts agree, though, that if you want to lose weight you have to consume fewer calories than you burn.

Cutting back on foods high in sugar and processed fats will go a long way toward trimming excess calories from your diet. Substitute plenty of vegetables and fruits, along with lean-protein foods, low-fat dairy products, legumes, and whole grains. Include small to moderate amounts of nuts, seeds, and unsaturated vegetable oils to get a healthy balance of fat. Other factors like exercise, stress management, and getting enough rest are also key to weight-loss success.

It's OK to try several diet plans until you find the one that works for you. Some experimentation may be needed to find the best pattern for you. You may be a person who wants everything spelled out—a point system you can count, meal by meal. Or you may be a person who just wants to work hard on cutting everything you eat into portions that are half the size you were used to. You may even want to try one of the more extreme diets for a brief period of time. A variety of dietary patterns can promote weight loss. But be aware that in the long run you will have to develop a workable, livable, sustainable, and satisfying diet. Chapter 4 presents some sample food pyramids that illustrate this point. By learning to eat well and customizing your diet to suit your personal nutrition needs, you can optimize your weight and avoid a frustrating up-and-down roller coaster ride.

4. FOODS THAT FIGHT DIABETES

Eating wisely is one of your most powerful weapons in the fight against diabetes. Both *what* you eat and *how much* you eat affect diabetes risk. If you take a close look at the typical American diet, it's easy to see why diabetes has reached epidemic proportions. Saturated fat and refined sugars make up about a quarter of the average person's caloric intake. Processed snack foods and other nutrient-poor foods—frequently in "supersize" portions—also feature prominently in many people's diets. Only a quarter of Americans eat the minimum recommended five-a-day vegetables and fruits. And most people get only half the dietary fiber needed for good health. Couple a diet like this with a sedentary lifestyle and you have a situation ripe for the development of type 2 diabetes.

If you're concerned that eating "wisely" means dieting and deprivation, you will be relieved to discover that nothing could be further from the truth. So what should you eat to defend yourself against diabetes? This chapter begins with an overview of the basics. Then we will help you put nutrition principles into practice with strategies for planning disease-fighting meals and snacks, both at home and when eating out.

In Search of the Optimal Diet

There is no known single optimal diet to prevent diabetes, which is probably good, since people have such different tastes and preferences. But much is known about individual foods and nutrients that raise or lower diabetes risk. For instance, whole grains, nuts, unsaturated fats, fiber, and magnesium have all been linked to a lower risk. Saturated and trans fats, refined carbohydrates, and high "glycemic load" foods (you'll learn more about the glycemic index and glycemic load starting on page 51), are associated with a higher chance of developing diabetes. This information provides a good starting point for building a healthy diet. Realize though, that when studies focus only on individual foods or nutrients—magnesium, or carbohydrate content, or chromium—they are probably only seeing small pieces of a puzzle, not the whole picture. Recently, researchers have begun to fit these pieces together by looking at dietary patterns that people practice in their everyday lives to determine which balance of different types of foods can best ward off diabetes.

In an effort to define the optimal diet for diabetes prevention, researchers at Harvard University studied the diets of more than 42,000 men for twelve years to see what protected against or predisposed a person to developing diabetes. Men who followed a "prudent" dietary pattern (higher in vegetables, fruit, fish, poultry, and whole grains) reduced their risk by 16 percent. On the other hand, men who followed a "Western" diet pattern (high in red meat, processed meat, French fries, high-fat dairy products, refined grains, sweets, and desserts) raised their risk of developing diabetes by nearly 60 percent. When the men with high "Western" diet scores were also sedentary, they doubled their risk for diabetes. Add obesity to the mix, and diabetes risk was raised more than elevenfold!

Another study of nearly 85,000 women found that a diet low in saturated and trans fat, low in glycemic load, and high in whole grains, was highly protective against diabetes. Women who ate this way reduced their diabetes risk by over half compared with women who had poor dietary scores. Women who ate wisely and who also were physically active, maintained a healthy weight, had moderate alcohol use, and abstained from smoking, reduced their diabetes risk by an astonishing 91 percent over the sixteen-year study period.

A Closer Look at Diet and Diabetes Risk

No single miracle food or dietary supplement will, by itself, prevent diabetes. However, the right overall balance of foods in your diet, and especially the overall *amount* of food, can offer substantial protection. The types and amounts of carbohydrate and fat eaten are especially important determinants of diabetes risk, because they are the foodstuffs that make up the majority of almost everyone's diet. Unfortunately, the media and the diet books have at best been confusing about carbohydrates, and at worst, downright inaccurate. So let's take a closer look at these nutrients and offer guidelines for making the best choices within each group.

CARBOHYDRATES—THE GOOD, THE BAD, AND THE GLYCEMIC INDEX

If you're confused about carbohydrates, you're not alone. Media hype over the years has flashed headlines stating anything from carbohydrates are our saviors to carbohydrates are the root of all evil. The truth is, the human body can adapt to a wide range of carbohydrate, fat, and protein intake. However, carbohydrate is the body's preferred fuel, the first fuel used when several are available, especially for the brain and nervous system. The body can survive with very little carbohydrate, but when there are no carbohydrates available and it has to turn to fat as the main energy source, this metabolic state is called "ketosis." The resulting chemicals formed, called ketones, can leave you feeling weak, tired, and irritable. According to guidelines issued by the National Academy of Sciences, most adults should consume at least 130 grams of carbohydrate per day to provide optimal fuel balance. The problem is that all carbohydrates are not created equal—and a diet high in the wrong kinds of carbohydrates sets the stage for diabetes, obesity, cardiovascular disease, and many other health problems.

Good Versus Bad Carbs

Throughout most of history, the only carbohydrate foods that were available were the wild roots, tubers, vegetables, fruits, and nuts that people foraged for. These foods were loaded with fiber and nutrients, and they were slowly digested and absorbed to provide a slow-release, sustained form of energy. With the advent of agriculture some 10,000 years ago, people began to cultivate grains such as wheat, rice, barley, oats, and corn. These

FIBER—THE MISSING LINK

Study after study supports the benefit of high-fiber foods in preventing obesity, diabetes, cardiovascular disease, and cancer. Yet most of the fiber—along with essential nutrients, antioxidants, and phytochemicals—is processed out of carbohydrate-rich foods today.

Viscous or *soluble* fibers found in foods like oats, legumes, barley, and many vegetables and fruits, may be especially beneficial to people at risk for diabetes. These foods are slowly digested and absorbed, resulting in lower blood glucose and insulin levels. They also create a sensation of fullness that helps prevent overeating.

The fiber in whole-grain breads and cereals also appears to protect against diabetes. One reason may be that these foods are rich in magnesium, which is associated with improved insulin sensitivity. Another reason may be that people who eat plenty of whole grains and other high-fiber foods tend to be thinner than people who eat diets high in refined carbohydrates.

How much fiber should you eat? Health experts recommend eating at least 25 to 35 grams daily (most people get only half this amount). Diets that provide up to 50 grams of fiber daily have been found to be even more beneficial for blood glucose, insulin, and cholesterol levels.

foods, which quickly became mainstays in the human diet, were consumed in their natural unprocessed forms. Whole, cracked, or coarsely ground grains were made into nutritious porridges or baked into hearty whole-grain breads. Vegetables and fruits were abundant and sugar was consumed only on rare occasions.

Fast-forward to the modern world and a very different picture emerges. The kinds of carbohydrates available in the food supply have changed dramatically—and definitely *not* for the better. The bulk of carbohydrate foods consumed today are highly refined and processed. Much of it is simple sugar—not only table sugar but candies, corn syrup, and sweet drinks. And it has very often been stripped of most of the nutrients and fiber.

For instance, the typical American diet currently supplies over thirty teaspoons of refined sugar daily! To make matters worse, 85 percent of all grains eaten today are refined—frequently in the form of white bread, white rice, processed breakfast cereals, snack chips, pretzels, cookies, pastries, and other nutrient-poor foods. Add to this the fact that foods like French fries and potato chips make up a substantial portion of our "vegetable" intake, and you can see the enormity of the problem.

The Glycemic Index

When you eat carbohydrate-containing foods, they are broken down in the stomach and intestine into sugar molecules, which are absorbed into the blood. Under the influence of insulin, the circulating blood sugar is then either burned for energy or stored away, mainly as fat, for later use when you aren't eating (such as overnight).

This brings up another problem with many of the carbohydrate foods that people eat today—they are very quickly digested and absorbed. A diet very high in quickly digested carbohydrates promotes more of a spike in blood glucose and insulin levels. Why is this a problem? Some research suggests that the rapid rises in glucose and insulin can contribute to diabetes, cardiovascular disease, and other health problems. In recent years, the "glycemic index" of foods has received a lot of attention; so let's take a look at what it is:

The *glycemic index* (GI) is a system developed in the 1980s to rank carbohydrates based on how much they raise blood sugar levels. High-GI foods are quickly digested and absorbed, producing a rapid rise in blood sugar and insulin levels. Low-GI foods, on the other hand, are slowly digested and absorbed, producing a smaller, more gradual rise in blood sugar and insulin levels.

The theory goes that because high-GI foods increase insulin demand and raise the workload of the pancreas, many years of eating a diet rich in high-GI foods can cause the pancreas to literally wear out, resulting in type 2 diabetes. Ongoing research will continue to shed light on this subject. But there is no doubt that different carbohydrates have different GIs, and the following table shows the glycemic index of some common foods compared to pure glucose, which has a GI of 100.

THE GLYCEMIC INDEX IN PERSPECTIVE.   While the GI is a useful dietary concept, the *total amount of calories and carbohydrate* are probably most important in planning a healthful diet. For instance, some sweets, junk foods, and other nutrient-poor foods have a low to moderate GI but are very high in calories, refined carbohydrate, and fat. And there is absolutely no doubt that taking in too many calories and gaining too much weight is the main cause of diabetes throughout the world. So in the next section, we discuss *glycemic load,* expanding on this notion that it's the total amount that matters most.

THE GLYCEMIC INDEX OF SOME COMMON FOODS			
Food	**GI**	**Food**	**GI**
Breakfast Cereals		Pita bread	57
All-Bran	42	Sourdough rye bread	53
Bran Chex	58	Cracked-wheat bread	58
Cheerios	74	White bread	70
Corn Flakes	81	*Vegetables*	
Grape Nuts Nuggets	71	Carrots	71
Oat Bran, Quaker	50	Corn, sweet	53
Oats, quick-cooking	66	Lima beans, baby	32
Oats, old-fashioned	58	Peas, green	48
Raisin Bran	61	Potatoes, baked	85
Rice Chex	89	Potatoes, French-fried	75
Breads		Potatoes, new	62
Bagel (white)	72	Sweet potatoes	54
Baguette	95	Tomato juice	38
Croissant	67	*Fruits*	
Kaiser roll	73	Apple	36
Linseed (flax) rye bread	55	Apricots, dried	31
Oat bran bread (50% oat bran)	47	Banana	52

THE GLYCEMIC INDEX OF SOME COMMON FOODS

FOOD	GI	FOOD	GI
Fruits (cont.)		*Grains*	
Cantaloupe	65	Barley	25
Cherries	22	Bulgur wheat	48
Grapefruit	25	Couscous	61
Grapes	46	Rice, long-grain, brown	55
Mango	51	Rice, long-grain, white	56
Orange	43	Rice, short-grain, white	88
Peach	28	Rice, wild	57
Pear	38	Wheat berries	41
Plum	39	*Pasta*	
Prunes	29	Egg fettuccine	40
Strawberries	40	Linguine	46
Watermelon	72	Spaghetti	44
Dairy		Spaghetti, whole wheat	37
Ice cream, low-fat	50	*Legumes*	
Milk, skim	32	Baked beans	48
Fruit yogurt, sugar-free	14	Black-eyed peas	42
Fruit yogurt, with sugar	33	Chickpeas	28
			(continued)

THE GLYCEMIC INDEX OF SOME COMMON FOODS			
FOOD	GI	FOOD	GI
Legumes (cont.)		*Sweets*	
Kidney beans	28	Chocolate	49
Lentils	30	Jellybeans	80
Lima beans, baby	32	Life Savers	70
Split peas	32	M&Ms (peanut)	33
Snack Foods		Mars Bars	62
Cheese puffs	74	Skittles	70
Peanuts	14	Snickers	55
Popcorn	55	Twix Cookie Bars (caramel)	44
Potato chips	54	Sucrose (white sugar)	65
Pretzels	83	Glucose	100

GLYCEMIC INDEX VERSUS GLYCEMIC LOAD.   To re-emphasize the main point: the glycemic index tells you how *quickly* a carbohydrate-containing food turns into sugar, but it doesn't tell you *how much* carbohydrate is in a serving of a food. This is where glycemic load comes in.

Glycemic load is a relatively new term that considers both the glycemic index *and* the amount of carbohydrate in a food. Carrots, for example, have a high GI, but carrots are low in total amount of carbohydrate, unless you eat massive amounts of carrots. So compared to other sources of carbohydrate, like bread, sweets, and potatoes, the glycemic *load* of carrots is relatively low. Sugary foods (candy, sodas, cookies, etc.) are very high in carbohydrate *and* tend to rank high on the glycemic index. In addition, because they taste sweet, you're likely to eat large amounts, so they can dramatically raise your glycemic load.

The bottom line is that if a food contains very little carbohydrate, it will not have much impact on blood sugar and insulin levels, regardless of its glycemic index. On the other hand, if a given meal has a high GI *and* high carbohydrate content, it will push the blood glucose, insulin (and body weight) up.

HOW TO LIGHTEN YOUR GLYCEMIC LOAD.   Generally speaking, and not surprisingly, foods that contribute most to the glycemic load are those that taste the best and "go down" the easiest. Those products include those made from white flour like breads, biscuits, muffins, and other baked goods; sugary foods like sodas, cakes, cookies, and candy; refined breakfast cereals; snack foods like chips and pretzels; and baked, mashed, and French fried potatoes. Since most of these are also high-calorie nutrient-poor foods, a high glycemic load is just one more reason to limit them.

Foods that are likely to contribute lower glycemic load include salad greens and nonstarchy vegetables; fruits; sweet potatoes; legumes; minimally processed whole grains such as thick-cut oatmeal, oat bran, long-grain brown rice, barley, and bulgur wheat; pasta; and dairy products. Since these are all nutrient-dense foods and most are rich in fiber, their low glycemic load is one more reason to include them in your diet often.

TIPS FOR LIGHTENING YOUR GLYCEMIC LOAD

- Include plenty of leafy greens and nonstarchy vegetables in meals.
- Choose hearty breads that contain high proportions of whole or cracked grains, stone-ground whole-wheat flour, oats, bran, and flaxseeds.
- Don't be fooled by "no-added-sugar" foods. Some foods are essentially all sugar to begin with, so none needs to be "added."
- Choose unrefined minimally processed cereals, such as old-fashioned oatmeal, oat bran, muesli, and All-Bran, and cereals made with psyllium.
- Substitute long-grain brown rice or wild rice for white rice.
- Substitute sweet potatoes or small new potatoes for baked, mashed, and French-fried potatoes.
- Replace part of the flour in baked goods with oat bran, rolled oats, wheat bran, or flaxmeal.

- Pair a sandwich with a cup of vegetable soup, fresh fruit, or salad instead of French fries, chips, or pretzels.
- Balance high-carbohydrate entrées like pasta and rice dishes with lower-carbohydrate side dishes like salads and nonstarchy vegetables.
- Snack on fruit, vegetables, popcorn, nuts (in moderation), and yogurt instead of chips, pretzels, cookies, and candy.
- Choose fruit- and dairy-based desserts instead of cakes, cookies, and flour-based desserts.

The Bottom Line on Carbs

In sum, there's nothing "wrong" with carbohydrates. In fact you can *reduce* your risk for diabetes, cardiovascular disease, cancer, and many other health problems by choosing more "good carbs" such as vegetables, fruits, legumes, and whole grains and by limiting foods that are high in sugar and white flour.

How much carbohydrate should you eat? Your personal carbohydrate needs will depend on your likes and dislikes, your activity level, health-risk profile, and weight-

SUGGESTED DAILY CARBOHYDRATE ALLOWANCES			
DAILY CALORIE INTAKE	CARBOHYDRATE INTAKE (40% OF CALORIES)	CARBOHYDRATE INTAKE (45% OF CALORIES)	CARBOHYDRATE INTAKE (50% OF CALORIES)
1,200	120 g	135 g	150 g
1,400	140 g	157 g	175 g
1,600	160 g	180 g	200 g
1,800	180 g	202 g	225 g
2,000	200 g	225 g	250 g
2,200	220 g	247 g	275 g

management goals. Most people who are overweight or at risk for diabetes or the metabolic syndrome would be wise to hold down their total caloric intake, and this often means limiting carbohydrate, as well as fat and protein. To put in some numbers on the recommendations, the table on page 56 lists the amount of carbohydrate that would be acceptable in diets of varying calorie levels. It is based on the fact that one gram of carbohydrate yields four calories.

SEPARATING FAT FROM FICTION

Just as all carbohydrates are not created equal, all fats are not equal either. Unfortunately, just as some people consider carbohydrates the enemy, others are under the false impression that all fats are bad and must be avoided at any cost. This misperception, which peaked in the 1990s, contributed to a whole new set of health problems—and a flood of fat-free foods that were as bad or worse than the foods they replaced.

Fat-Free Foods—What Went Wrong?

Over the past couple of decades, low-fat diets have been widely recommended for treating both diabetes and heart disease. The main point is that too much of the fat in people's diets has traditionally been *saturated* fat, which raises cholesterol levels and may promote cardiovascular disease. In recent years, though, it has become apparent that for many people, a low-fat diet can actually make things worse. How can this be? The low-fat diet in its original form was very different from the low-fat diet of today.

The low-fat diet of the 1970s and early '80s was composed primarily of vegetables, fruits, whole grains, legumes, lean meats, skinless poultry, fish, and low-fat dairy products. So it was higher in healthy carbohydrates and protein, high in fiber, and naturally low in calories. In other words, it promoted weight loss. The diet was also packed with health-promoting nutrients, antioxidants, and phytochemicals.

As low-fat diets caught on in the 1980s, though, manufacturers began to develop new kinds of low-fat foods. Some of these, such as leaner meats, lower-fat dairy products, and low-fat mayonnaise, were a real boon to the fat-fighter. Others, such as fat-free cookies, candies, pastries, and snack chips, were loaded with sugar and white flour. This started the downfall of the low-fat diet. As these foods flooded the marketplace, the nutritional value of many people's diets went down—and their caloric intake and glycemic load went up.

On the plus side, our increased fat awareness over the past few decades means that many more people have become aware of the harmful effects of saturated fat on their cholesterol levels, and many have reduced their saturated fat intake, a trend that seems to correlate with decreased cardiovascular disease. What's wrong with this? Well, just holding back saturated fat isn't enough. In fact, reliance on the kind of high-sugar carbohydrates discussed above can more than erase the benefits of reducing fat. Again, the *total* number of calories in the typical American diet is out of control.

Is High Fat Any Better?

In recent years, there has been a proliferation of high-protein and high-fat diets. The Atkins diet is the prototype. Many books even recommend a steady diet of saturated-fat meats, bacon, pork rinds, butter, and cream. We do *not* recommend this. Instead, we recommend making your food choices with moderation and common sense. Build your diet around both good carbs *and* good fats. Because one thing is very clear: different fats have very different health benefits. The next section will help explain this. Chapter 3 will sum up the pros and cons of high-fat, high-protein versus low-fat, high-carb diets for weight loss.

Fats to Choose and Fats to Avoid

Recommendations regarding fat intake to improve health boil down to some very simple guidelines:

- Avoid saturated fats and transfats.
- Choose polyunsaturated and monounsaturated fats.

Saturated fats (found in high-fat meats and dairy products) and trans fats (found in hydrogenated vegetable oils) increase levels of "bad" (LDL) cholesterol and foster the development of heart disease. So they're the "bad guys" of fat. Polyunsaturated and monounsaturated fats (except for trans fats), on the other hand, actually lower LDL cholesterol. Found in fish, vegetable oils, nuts, and seeds, they're the "good guys."

And of the polyunsaturated fats, the omega-3 type deserves special mention because it can dramatically reduce the risk of cardiovascular disease and may thwart a number of other health problems, Since most people's diets are woefully deficient in this essential fat, it is well worth making the effort to increase your intake (as the following tips show, this is very easy to do).

All this may seem complicated if you don't know your saturated fats from your monos and polys. For more information about dietary fats see the inset below entitled "Dietary

Fats 101". If you want to cut right to the chase, just follow the simple strategies outlined below and you will automatically get a healthy balance of fat.

HOW TO GET A HEALTHY BALANCE OF FATS

- Choose lean meats and low-fat dairy products. This will greatly reduce your intake of harmful saturated fat.
- Have fish (especially oily fish like salmon and sardines) at least twice a week. This will supply essential omega-3 fatty acids.
- Use canola, soybean, olive, and walnut oils for cooking and salads. This will supply a healthy balance of monounsaturated and polyunsaturated fats, including omega-3 fat.
- Choose mayonnaise, salad dressings, and soft or "trans-free" margarines made from canola, soybean, olive, and walnut oils. This will also supply a healthy balance of monounsaturated and polyunsaturated fats.

DIETARY FATS 101

SATURATED FAT.

Saturated fats are associated with insulin resistance and a higher diabetes risk. Saturated fats also elevate LDL (bad) blood cholesterol levels and raise the risk for cardiovascular disease. Fatty meats; high-fat dairy products like whole milk, butter, cream, full-fat cheese, ice cream, and full-fat sour cream; and coconuts are all high in saturated fat. Saturated fat is often easy to spot because it is solid at room temperature (like the fat around a steak, in a strip of bacon, or a stick of butter).

TRANS FAT.

This fat is formed when liquid vegetable oils are hydrogenated to make them more solid. Trans fats behave like saturated fats in the body and may in fact be even worse for your health. Trans fats are linked to insulin resistance and diabetes. One study found that a diet high in trans fat increased diabetes risk by 31 percent. Like saturated fats, trans fats also raise LDL (bad) cholesterol. In addition, they lower HDL (good) cholesterol, posing a dual risk for cardiovascular disease.

Trans fats are found in partially hydrogenated vegetable oils, vegetable shortenings, and hard margarines. Commercial bakery items, processed snack foods, fried foods, and other foods that contain shortening or hydrogenated vegetable oils are also big offenders.

MONOUNSATURATED FAT.

Popularized by the heart-healthy "Mediterranean diet," monounsaturated fats have become a staple in many people's diets. Olive oil is the best-known source of monounsaturated fat, but canola oil, avocadoes, and most nuts are rich in monounsaturated fats as well. While monounsaturates are a healthful choice, remember that they are still a concentrated source of calories, so include them in your diet with your weight-management goals in mind.

POLYUNSATURATED FAT.

Two types of polyunsaturated fats, known as *omega-6* and *omega-3,* are essential for life. The ratio of these two fatty acids in your diet is also important because they have very powerful and very opposing effects on the body. Researchers believe that humans evolved on a diet that provided about equal amounts of omega-6 and omega-3 fats. Modern diets, however, which are based on grain-fed meats and hydrogenated oils, supply up to twenty times as much omega-6 as omega-3 fat. This imbalance favors the development of cardiovascular disease and may also promote cancer and inflammatory and autoimmune diseases like rheumatoid arthritis and lupus.

How can you get more omega-3 fats? Fatty fish is the best source of some especially potent omega-3 fats known as EPA and DHA. Among plant foods, flaxseeds and flax oil are the most concentrated sources. Canola oil, walnuts, and soy are also good sources of this essential fat. Health experts recommend about 1.5 to 2 grams of omega-3s from plant sources daily, and 4 to 5 grams of omega-3 fat from fish weekly.

■ Include healthy high-fat foods such as avocadoes, nuts, and seeds in your diet regularly, keeping your weight-management goals in mind.

■ Pass up processed foods like biscuits, croissants, crackers, donuts, cookies, snack chips, and fried foods made with hydrogenated vegetable oils or shortening. This will curtail your intake of harmful trans fat.

OMEGA-3 CONTENT OF SELECTED FOODS	
FOOD	OMEGA-3 FAT
Salmon (3 ounces)	1.5 g
Sardines (3 ounces)	1.59 g
Flaxseed oil (1 teaspoon)	2.5 g
Flaxseeds (1 tablespoon)	1.61 g
Canola oil (1 tablespoon)	1.27 g
Walnuts (2 tablespoons)	1.36 g
Walnut oil (1 tablespoon)	1.42 g
Soybean oil (1 tablespoon)	0.93 g
Tofu, firm (4 ounces)	0.66 g
Roasted soynuts (¼ cup)	0.73 g

- Substitute flaxmeal for part of the flour in baked goods for an omega-3 boost.
- Choose omega-3 enriched eggs when you use whole eggs.

The Fat-Calorie Connection

The contribution of fat to total calorie intake cannot be overemphasized. Once again, fat has 9 calories per gram, so it is a very concentrated source of calories compared with carbohydrate (4 calories per gram) and protein (4 calories per gram). This is why high-fat meats and dairy products frequently have twice the calories of their low-fat counterparts. This is also why you double the calories in potatoes by making them into French fries, triple the calories in pasta by tossing it in cream sauce, and increase calories tenfold by making cabbage into coleslaw. The moral of this story is be careful of fats in your diet. To

SUGGESTED DAILY FAT ALLOWANCES				
DAILY CALORIE INTAKE	FAT INTAKE (20% OF CALORIES)	FAT INTAKE (25% OF CALORIES)	FAT INTAKE (30% OF CALORIES)	FAT INTAKE (35% OF CALORIES)
1,200	27 g	33 g	40 g	47 g
1,400	31 g	39 g	47 g	54 g
1,600	35 g	44 g	53 g	62 g
1,800	40 g	50 g	60 g	70 g
2,000	44 g	55 g	67 g	78 g
2,200	49 g	61 g	73 g	85 g

put things in perspective, the table above lists the amount of fat that would be acceptable in diets of varying calorie levels.

WHERE DOES PROTEIN FIT IN?

Very little information is available regarding protein intake and diabetes risk. Protein in a meal does not have much effect on blood glucose level, since it stimulates both insulin and the counter-insulin hormone glucagon. Some studies show that red meat and processed meats are associated with a higher risk of diabetes, but the saturated fat in these foods is a likely contributing factor. Other studies show that substituting protein for some of the carbohydrate in your diet can lower blood sugar, insulin, and triglyceride levels, possibly reducing diabetes risk.

An important point to bear in mind is that most foods called "high-protein" are in fact high-fat, and most diets called "high-protein" are in fact high-fat. A tender, juicy steak is the best example: much more fat than protein.

What's a person to do? The wisest course is to choose lean meats and skinless poultry since this will limit your intake of saturated fats and trim excess calories. Have fish at least twice a week to supply beneficial omega-3 fats. And substitute legumes and other vegetarian alternatives for meat often, as these foods supply fiber, nutrients, and phytochemicals that can help fight diabetes.

How much protein should you eat? One-half gram per pound of ideal body weight is a good starting point. Athletes and people over age fifty may need additional protein to meet their needs. People who are trying to lose weight usually benefit from additional protein as well. On the other hand, people with certain medical conditions such as kidney or liver disease may need to eat less protein. A registered dietitian can help you decide how much protein is right for you. Chapter 6 provides more information for choosing the most healthful protein choices.

A Word about Alcohol

Many studies have shown that alcohol, when consumed in moderation, reduces the risk of heart disease. Now it appears that alcohol may help prevent diabetes as well. How could this happen? By reducing insulin resistance. Studies show that light-to-moderate alcohol consumption (one to two drinks per day) is associated with improved insulin sensitivity, lower blood glucose and insulin levels, and higher HDL (good) cholesterol. Since high blood insulin levels may be a risk for cardiovascular disease, the insulin lowering potential of alcohol could partly explain how alcohol reduces the risk for heart disease.

A word of caution is always in order before considering using alcohol for "medicinal purposes." The most important caution, of course, is alcohol abuse—we need not emphasize the medical and social devastation caused by alcoholism. Studies have shown that the medical benefits of moderate alcohol intake are negated at exactly the level that motor vehicle accidents occur. Alcohol can also react adversely with a variety of medications and can occasionally cause hypoglycemia in people who use insulin or pills to control diabetes. People with liver disease should not consume alcohol. For these reasons, consult with your health-care practitioner about how alcohol use fits into your own particular situation.

Why One Diet Does Not Fit All

This chapter has covered the basic principles of eating to prevent diabetes and promote optimal health. It's important, though, to take this information and customize it to fit

SWEETS & JUNK FOODS

NUTS & SEEDS, UNSATURATED FATS

LEAN MEATS, POULTRY, FISH, EGGS, SOY, LEGUMES

LOW-FAT DAIRY OR SOY MILK, CHEESE, YOGURT

NONSTARCHY VEGETABLES & FRUITS

UNPROCESSED GRAINS & CEREALS, COARSE-GRAIN BREADS, STARCHY VEGETABLES

High-Carbohydrate Food Pyramid

This pyramid gets most of its calories from carbohydrate. It is well suited for very active people who are not concerned with losing weight.

your own needs because no one diet is good for everyone. People have different food preferences, lifestyles, metabolisms, and physical activity levels. For instance, someone who is very physically active and/or has a high metabolic rate will most likely benefit from a diet that is higher in carbohydrate than someone who is less active and/or has a lower metabolic rate. Some experimentation will probably be necessary to find the diet pattern that works best for you. A registered dietitian can help customize your diet based on your medical history and unique nutritional needs. Pages 64–66 present some sample food pyramids that illustrate a range of possible diet patterns.

In summary, certain fundamentals should take center stage when planning your diabetes-fighting diet. The single most important factor in preventing diabetes is without question

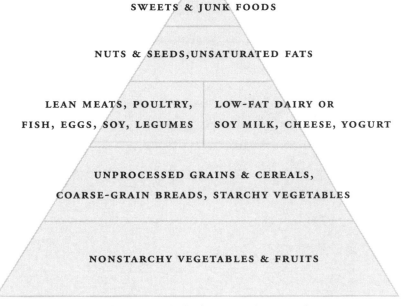

SWEETS & JUNK FOODS

NUTS & SEEDS, UNSATURATED FATS

LEAN MEATS, POULTRY, FISH, EGGS, SOY, LEGUMES

LOW-FAT DAIRY OR SOY MILK, CHEESE, YOGURT

UNPROCESSED GRAINS & CEREALS, COARSE-GRAIN BREADS, STARCHY VEGETABLES

NONSTARCHY VEGETABLES & FRUITS

Moderate-Carbohydrate Food Pyramid

This pyramid contains a moderate amount of carbohydrate and is suited for people who do not get much exercise or tend to gain weight easily.

restriction of total caloric intake to maintain normal body weight. Fats should be unsaturated, grains should be unrefined and minimally processed, meats should be lean, and dairy products low in fat. Vegetables and fruits should be abundant and added sugar should be limited. Beyond these basic guidelines, a variety of ranges for carbohydrates, protein, and fat can comprise a healthy diet—provided you consume the right amount of calories to sustain a healthy body weight. These same dietary principles will also help protect against cardiovascular disease, cancer, and many other common health problems.

SWEETS & JUNK FOODS

NUTS & SEEDS,UNSATURATED FATS

UNPROCESSED GRAINS & CEREALS,
COARSE-GRAIN BREADS, STARCHY VEGETABLES

LEAN MEATS, POULTRY,
FISH, EGGS, SOY, LEGUMES

LOW-FAT DAIRY OR
SOY MILK, CHEESE, YOGURT

NONSTARCHY VEGETABLES & FRUITS

Moderately Low-Carb Food Pyramid

This pyramid is lowest in carbohydrate and highest in protein. It emphasizes healthier food choices than most of the high-protein, low-carb fad diets that are out there today, and it is not as extreme. This pattern might be helpful to someone who finds weight loss difficult on higher-carbohydrate diets.

5. THE PREDIABETES PANTRY

The previous chapter illustrated how specific foods and dietary patterns can either prevent or promote the development of diabetes. This chapter will help you put these principles into practice so you can make your diet work for you—instead of against you. The basic concept is not rocket science: *What you don't have on your shelf, you won't eat.* So every time you shop, you are pretty much determining what you'll be eating until you shop again. Read on to discover how to choose the best diabetes-fighting foods to create simple, delicious, and satisfying meals and snacks.

Stocking Your Pantry

If you keep your pantry, refrigerator, and freezer stocked with the right foods, you will always have the makings of a healthful and delicious meal or snack on hand. Here are some foods to stock up on.

FRESH VEGETABLES, FRUITS, AND PRODUCE

Generous amounts of vegetables and fruits are at the very heart of a diabetes prevention diet. In fact, virtually no one has anything bad to say about vegetables and fruits—they will help you keep your weight in check and also protect against heart disease, cancer, and many other health problems. Plan to fill at least half of your plate with vegetables and fruits at each meal.

To keep calories and carbs under control, emphasize low-carbohydrate nonstarchy vegetables like broccoli, green beans, Brussels sprouts, cabbage, cauliflower, summer squash, greens, and salad vegetables. Think of starchy vegetables like potatoes, corn, baked beans, lima beans, and peas as bread or rice substitutes and include them in your diet as your carbohydrate and calorie budgets allow.

- Assorted fresh seasonal vegetables and fruits
- Prewashed salad greens
- Prewashed spinach
- Prewashed collard, turnip, mustard greens, and kale
- Baby carrots
- Fresh matchstick carrots
- Preshredded coleslaw mix
- Broccoli slaw
- Cherry and grape tomatoes

EATING NUTS EVERY DAY MAY
KEEP DIABETES AWAY

Numerous studies have shown that nuts protect against heart disease. Now it appears that these crunchy morsels may fight diabetes as well. In a recent study, researchers who tracked the diets of over 83,000 women found that women who ate an ounce of nuts at least five times a week were 27 percent less likely to develop diabetes than women who rarely ate nuts. Eating peanut butter regularly was even associated with a 21-percent lower risk of developing diabetes.

How might nuts protect against diabetes? The fiber and magnesium in nuts help maintain lower blood glucose and insulin levels. In addition, nuts are high in polyunsaturated and monounsaturated fats, which may help prevent insulin resistance. Other constituents of nuts, such as antioxidants, phytochemicals, and protein, may play a role in diabetes prevention as well.

This sort of study isn't final proof, of course: Just because there is an *association* between eating nuts and a reduced risk of diabetes does not prove that it's the nuts that protect. There may be other habits, dietary or otherwise, that protect people who also eat nuts. Also, a word of warning: A quarter cup of nuts contains about 200 calories, so it's important to find ways to *substitute* nuts for other foods such as snack chips and sweets. This way you can keep calories under control and improve the quality of your diet.

- Ready-cut vegetables for snacking and cooking
- Precut fresh fruits
- Avocadoes (use moderately if you are watching your weight)
- Crushed garlic and ginger
- Assorted nuts and seeds (use moderately if you are watching your weight)
- Tofu

BREADS, CEREALS, AND GRAINS

Choosing whole-grain products instead of refined versions is a top diabetes prevention strategy. Loaded with fiber, nutrients, and phytochemicals, whole-grain foods can also help keep your weight in check. Just remember that breads and grain products are concentrated sources of carbohydrate (though not nearly as high as sweets and desserts), so it's important to watch portions if you need to limit carbohydrates and calories.

- Hearty 100 percent whole-grain breads, bagels, and burger buns that include ingredients like stone-ground whole-wheat flour, oats, oat bran, wheat berries, and cracked wheat, whole rye, and flaxseeds.
- Lower-carb, high-fiber breads. A wide array of sandwich breads, and burger and hot dog buns are available with about half the carbs of regular bread. Note that some "light" and lower-carb breads are made with predominately white flour with added fibers, so look for brands that contain whole-grain ingredients to get the most nutrition.
- Whole-grain English muffins.
- Whole-grain pita bread.
- Whole-wheat flour tortillas.

WHOLE GRAINS—HOW TO FIND THE "REAL THING"

Choosing 100 percent *whole-grain* products instead of refined versions can reduce your diabetes risk. Unfortunately, finding these fiber-rich products can be a real chore because products like "natural grain bread" and "golden wheat crackers" may contain far more refined white flour than whole grains. Here are some clues that can help you hone in on the real thing:

- Whole wheat, or another whole grain such as whole rye or oats should be listed as the *first* ingredient.
- Check out the ingredient list for other fiber-rich ingredients like wheat bran, oat bran, wheat berries, bulgur wheat, wheat germ, and flax.
- Avoid products that list "wheat" or "enriched wheat" as the first ingredient, as these are other names for refined wheat.
- Whole-grain products will have at least 2 grams of fiber per slice of bread, ounce of crackers, or ounce of cereal.

- Corn tortillas. Choose thin corn tortillas, which have about 25 to 35 calories and 6 to 8 grams of carbohydrate per tortilla instead of thick tortillas, which have up to twice this amount.
- Chapati (a whole-wheat Indian flatbread similar to a tortilla).
- Whole-grain crackers (like Wasa Bread, Rye Krisp, Kavli, Rye Vita, Ak-mak, and reduced-fat Triscuits).
- Whole-wheat pasta.
- Wheat-blend pasta. Pastas made with part whole-wheat and part white flour are available in most grocery stores. These products can be a good way to transition to 100 percent whole-grain pasta.
- Whole-grain cereals like old-fashioned oatmeal, oat bran, All-Bran, Wheat Chex, Bran Chex, Shredded Wheat, Raisin Bran, Uncle Sam Cereal, Kashi, Health Valley, and Wheetabix (look for at least 5 grams of fiber per 2-ounce serving).
- Whole-grains like barley, brown rice, wild rice, bulgur wheat, quinoa, and whole-wheat couscous.
- Air-popped or light microwave popcorn.
- Whole-grain and buckwheat pancake mixes.

HOW WHOLE GRAINS FIGHT DIABETES

People who eat whole grains are less likely to develop diabetes. What is it about whole grains that confers protection? These foods are rich in fiber, magnesium, antioxidants, and beneficial phytochemicals that may help the body process carbohydrates more efficiently.

One study also suggested that insulin sensitivity is improved. Investigators found that people who made no other dietary changes except to substitute whole-grain breads, cereals, rice, and pasta for refined versions lowered their fasting insulin levels by 10 percent over a six-week study period. They were also less hungry between meals than people who ate the refined versions of these foods, and they actually preferred the whole-grain diet to the refined version.

CANNED AND JARRED FOODS

- Unsweetened applesauce
- Artichoke hearts and bottoms (drain marinated hearts before using)
- Dill and sugar-free sweet pickles (in moderation—they are high in sodium)
- Dried beans such as black, kidney, pinto, navy, garbanzo, black-eyed peas, and chili beans (draining and rinsing removes about 40 percent of the sodium)
- Fruits canned in juice
- Hot peppers
- Olives
- Peanut butter and nut butters (they are high in calories so use in moderation)
- Sugar-free and low-sugar fruit pie fillings
- Roasted red bell peppers
- Soups—chicken, turkey, or beef with vegetables; vegetarian vegetable; bean; lentil; split pea; tomato; and low-fat cream soups
- Sun-dried tomatoes packed in olive oil (drain before using)
- Spaghetti and marinara sauce (look for brands with little or no added sugar or fat)
- Tomatoes, stewed tomatoes, tomato sauce, tomato paste
- Tomato juice
- Tuna, salmon, crab, sardines, anchovies
- Vegetable juice cocktail

CONDIMENTS AND SEASONINGS

- Anchovies and anchovy paste
- Capers
- Spice blends such as Italian seasoning; fines herbes; herbs de Provence; curry paste (curry spices mixed with canola oil, ground lentils, and other ingredients); Mrs. Dash; Lawry's Pinch of Herbs; lemon pepper: and Cajun, Greek, and jerk seasonings
- Horseradish

- Hot sauce
- Jams and preserves (choose low-sugar and all-fruit types)
- Ketchup and barbecue sauce (these condiments are high in sugar so use in moderation). Reduced sugar versions are now available as well.
- Lemon juice
- Low-fat and fat-free mayonnaise
- Mustard
- Reduced-sodium soy sauce
- Salad dressings, nonfat and light (compare labels for sugar content)
- Salad dressings, regular (choose those made with canola, olive, soybean, or walnut oil and use in moderation if you are watching your weight)
- Salsa and picante sauce
- Packaged dry sauce mixes such as Alfredo, creamy tomato, cheese, and pesto (to trim calories from creamy sauces, omit the butter or margarine and use low-fat milk or evaporated skim milk instead of regular milk)
- Vinegars—balsamic, red wine, white wine, sherry, apple cider, raspberry, and others
- Worcestershire sauce

FATS AND OILS

Be aware that all oils have 120 calories per tablespoon. Full-fat margarines and mayonnaise contain 90 to 100 calories per tablespoon. Use these products sparingly if you are watching your weight.

- Canola oil (good source of omega-3 fat)
- Extra-virgin olive oil
- Soybean oil (good source of omega-3 fat)
- Walnut oil (good source of omega-3 fat)
- Sesame oil
- Nonstick vegetable oil cooking sprays
- Light trans-free margarine
- Regular margarine (use moderately—high in calories)
- Light butter and light whipped butter (high in saturated fat, use in moderation)

- Nonfat and light mayonnaise
- Regular mayonnaise (use moderately—high in calories)

Dairy Products

- Low-fat and nonfat cottage cheese
- Low-fat and nonfat ricotta cheese
- Low-fat and nonfat cream cheese
- Neufchâtel (light cream cheese)
- Soft-curd farmer cheese
- Reduced-fat feta cheese
- Parmesan cheese (Parmesan is a full-fat cheese, but a little bit goes a long way, making this an acceptable choice.)
- Reduced-fat and nonfat mozzarella, Cheddar, Monterey Jack, provolone, and Swiss (Tip: reduced-fat cheeses work best in recipes in which you need a cheese that melts well; nonfat brands work fine atop a salad or in a cold dish)
- Soy cheese
- Nonfat (skim) and 1% low-fat milk
- Nonfat and low-fat buttermilk
- Evaporated skim or low-fat milk (use to lighten coffee or as a cream substitute in sauces, quiches, and other dishes)
- Instant nonfat dry milk powder
- Plain nonfat and low-fat yogurt
- Flavored nonfat and low-fat yogurt (choose "light" and sugar-free brands to cut calories by almost half)
- Nonfat and light sour cream

Eggs

- Fat-free egg substitutes (like Egg Beaters)
- Egg whites
- Omega-3 enriched eggs—these eggs come from hens that eat a diet enriched with ingredients like flaxseed, marine algae, and fishmeal (most people can eat four to seven egg yolks per week: ask your dietitian or physician to make a recommendation for your specific needs)

DAIRY PRODUCTS FIGHT INSULIN RESISTANCE SYNDROME

A recent study adds the metabolic syndrome (also known as insulin resistance syndrome) to the list of health problems that dairy products may protect against. Researchers who examined the eating habits of more than 3,000 men and women found that overweight people who consumed the most dairy products were about 70 percent less likely to develop metabolic syndrome than were people who consumed few dairy products. Each additional daily serving of dairy was associated with a 21-percent lower risk of developing the syndrome over the ten-year study period. People who ate plenty of dairy products were also less likely to gain unwanted pounds over the duration of the study.

How might dairy products offer this protection? The carbohydrate in milk (lactose) is slowly absorbed, which helps control blood sugar and insulin levels. The protein in milk helps fill you up, which may help keep your weight in check. In addition, the calcium, potassium, and magnesium in dairy foods likely play a role in preventing insulin resistance. These nutrients are beneficial for reducing blood pressure, which is commonly associated with insulin resistance. In fact, a major study found that adding two servings of low-fat dairy products to the daily diet boosted the blood pressure lowering benefits of a healthy high-fiber diet.

Dietary trends over the past several decades show that people are substituting more sodas and processed snack foods for dairy products like milk and yogurt. Experts believe that this change in dietary pattern may play a role in the dramatic upsurge of obesity and insulin resistance syndrome seen in recent years.

MEAT, POULTRY, AND SEAFOOD

Including some protein in meals and snacks will make them more filling and satisfying—important considerations for people who are watching their weight. Of course, not all high-protein foods are alike, so be sure to choose well-trimmed meats and skinless poultry to keep calories and saturated fat at a minimum. Bear in mind that processed meats like luncheon meats and hot dogs are high in sodium; so eat these foods less often. Be sure to eat fish at least twice a week and substitute high-protein vegetarian alternatives for meat often.

- Skinless chicken and turkey
- Ground turkey (look for ground turkey that is at least 95 percent lean)
- Beef round, eye of round, round tip, top sirloin, London Broil, flat half brisket
- Ground beef (look for ground beef that is 93 to 96 percent lean)
- Pork tenderloin, loin roast, sirloin chops, loin chops
- Ham (look for ham that is at least 95 percent lean)
- Extra-lean turkey bacon (Tip: for a crisp texture, cook turkey bacon in a microwave oven; turkey bacon that is cooked in a skillet will have a chewy texture)
- Canadian bacon
- Smoked sausage and kielbasa (look for products that are at least 95 to 97 percent lean)
- Luncheon meats and hot dogs (look for products that are at least 95 to 97 percent lean)
- Assorted fresh fish and shellfish (choose oily fish like salmon, sardines, and herring often for their healthful omega-3 fatty acids
- Canned tuna, salmon, and crab packed in spring water or pouches
- Sardines packed in mustard or tomato sauce
- Frozen shrimp

VEGETARIAN MEAT ALTERNATIVES

Lots of people have turned to vegetarian diets, for all sorts of reasons. And planned properly, a vegetarian diet is a very healthy way to eat. So try substituting these foods for meat often, because they are low in saturated fats, cholesterol-free, and rich in health-promoting nutrients and phytochemicals that are not present in meats.

- Tofu. Substitute crumbled firm tofu for part or all of the eggs in egg salad; add crumbled tofu to scrambled eggs or sprinkle it over a salad as you would cheese. Substitute cubed firm or extra-firm tofu for meat in stir-fry dishes; use soft and silken tofu as a base for dips, sauces, and smoothies.
- Tofu hamburger and frozen recipe crumbles. These mildly seasoned bits of tofu or vegetable protein look like crumbled ground beef and can substitute for part or all of the ground beef in many recipes. Two cups of tofu hamburger is the equivalent of one pound of ground beef.

- Texturized vegetable protein (TVP). These small nuggets, made from soybeans, look similar to grape nuts. They are rehydrated with water or broth and then used in recipes as you would tofu hamburger or recipes crumbles.
- Veggie burgers.
- Vegetarian lunchmeats, hot dogs, and sausages. These products are made from soy and other vegetable proteins. Like processed meats, these products can be high in sodium and may contain artificial ingredients so use them less often than other vegetarian alternatives.
- Legumes (dried beans, peas, and lentils). Legumes are loaded with cholesterol-lowering fiber and nutrients and have a very gentle effect on blood sugar compared with carbohydrate-rich foods like potatoes and bread. Purchase dried or canned legumes and use in a variety of recipes from dips and spreads to casseroles, soups, and salads.
- Nuts, peanut butter, and nut butters. A quarter cup of nuts or two tablespoons of peanut/nut butter contains as much protein as one ounce of meat, and close to 200 calories; use moderately if you are watching your weight.

DELI

- Rotisserie chicken (remove the skin)
- Hummus
- Tabbouleh
- Low-fat cole slaw, macaroni salad, pasta salad, potato salad
- Sliced turkey breast, roast beef, lean corned beef, lean ham (limit processed meats due to high sodium content)

FROZEN FOODS

- Veggie burgers
- Vegetarian sausage and bacon
- Frozen dinners such as Healthy Choice
- Plain frozen vegetables

- Plain frozen fruits
- Whole-grain frozen waffles
- Frozen fruit juice bars
- Low-sugar Fudgesicles and Popsicles
- Low-fat ice cream and frozen yogurt (see the inset on page 231 for more on choosing ice cream)
- Nonfat and light whipped topping

BAKING INGREDIENTS

To prevent rancidity, be sure to store products like whole-grain flour, flaxmeal, and wheat germ in the refrigerator or freezer.

- Flaxseeds. Loaded with healthful omega-3 fats, flaxseeds can be ground in a blender or coffee grinder into flax meal, which can replace up to 25 percent of the flour in muffins, quick breads, and other recipes. (Note: Flax experts recommend limiting intake to 1 tablespoon of ground flaxseed per day until more is known about the health effects of consuming larger amounts.)
- Rolled oats and oat bran. Replace part of the flour in muffins, quick breads, and other recipes with oatmeal or oat bran for a fiber and nutrition boost.
- Oat flour. Ground from whole-grain oats, oat flour lends a slightly sweet flavor and a tender texture to baked goods, reducing the need for fat and sugar. Rich in fiber and nutrients, oat flour also improves the nutritional profile of foods when you substitute it for part of the white flour in recipes. These qualities make oat flour a natural for healthy baking. Oat flour can replace up to half of the flour in products like muffins, quick breads, cakes, and cookies. This product can be purchased in natural food stores and some grocery stores. Or make your own oat flour by grinding quick-cooking oats in a blender or food processor. One cup of oats will make about ¾ cup of flour.
- Wheat bran. Give a fiber boost to muffins and quick breads by replacing part of the flour with wheat bran.
- Wheat germ. Loaded with vitamin E, minerals, and B vitamins. Replace up to 25 percent of the flour in baked goods with this supernutritious product.
- Whole-wheat flour. Use to replace part or all of the white flour in homemade yeast breads.

- White whole-wheat flour. A lighter-tasting alternative to regular whole-wheat flour. This product can be used in yeast breads and quick breads, muffins, pancakes, and many other recipes.
- Whole-wheat pastry flour. Made especially for products like muffins, quick breads, cookies, and pancakes, this product has a lightly sweet flavor and softer texture than regular whole-wheat flour. It does not contain enough gluten to work in most yeast breads though.
- Whole-grain and buckwheat pancake mixes.

SWEETS AND DESSERTS

Satisfying the sweet tooth can be a real challenge when watching carbs and calories. Here are some of the better choices to look for in your grocery store. You should be aware that some sugar-free products are quite high in calories and fat and may not be better choices than the "real thing." The insets on pages 79–82 provide more information about the various sweeteners that are used to sweeten sugar-free foods.

THE SCOOP ON SUGAR ALCOHOLS

An increasing number of "sugar-free" products are sweetened with sugar alcohols. Many sugar alcohols are easily spotted in the ingredients list of food labels because their names end in –ol. Sorbitol, maltitol, and xylitol are some examples. Hydrogenated starch hydrolosyates and isomalt are examples of sugar alcohols that do not have the –ol suffix.

Sugar alcohols are made from ingredients like beet sugar and cornstarch, which have been chemically rearranged to resist digestion. As a result, sugar alcohols are poorly absorbed, have a minimal effect on blood sugar levels, and supply about half the calories of regular sugar. The caveat is: If too much is eaten, sugar alcohols can cause bloating, gas, and have a laxative effect. Furthermore, many sugar alcohol-sweetened products save you few or no calories—which is why they often bear labels that state "not for weight control." The bottom line is always read labels—and first and foremost, be sure to compare calories.

- ■ Sugar-free pudding mixes
- ■ Sugar-free gelatin
- ■ Sugar-free Fudgesicles
- ■ Sugar-free Popsicles
- ■ 100 percent fruit and juice bars
- ■ Fruits canned in natural juice
- ■ Unsweetened applesauce
- ■ Low-fat ice cream and frozen yogurt (see the inset on page 231 for more on choosing ice cream)
- ■ Plain, unfilled lady fingers (top with fresh fruit and some light whipped topping)
- ■ Dark chocolate (high in calories, use in moderation)
- ■ Sugar-free hot chocolate
- ■ Light (sugar-free or low-sugar) pie fillings
- ■ Nonfat and light whipped toppings
- ■ Oatmeal cookies made with nonhydrogenated fats (high in carbs, eat in moderation)

SUGAR SUBSTITUTES

In a quest to trim carbs and calories from recipes, many people turn to sugar substitutes. However, when using these products in recipes, it's important to understand that sugar adds more than just sweetness. For instance, sugar adds texture and tenderness, helps retain moisture, and promotes the browning of baked goods. For this reason, replacing all of the sugar in baked goods like cakes, cookies and muffins with an artificial sweetener can result in a very disappointing (pale, rubbery, and dry) product. This is why some of the recipes in this book do contain some real sugar. On the other hand, products like pies, fruit crisps, puddings, and gelatin desserts more easily adapt to using sugar substitutes. A wide variety of sugar substitutes are available to choose from. Here is a brief description of some of these products and their suitability for recipes.

ACESULFAME-K.

Sold under the brand name Sunette, acesulfame-K has a pleasant flavor and leaves no bitter aftertaste. This product is heat stable, so can be used in cooked foods.

ASPARTAME.

Also known as NutraSweet and Equal. Aspartame is made of two amino acids (the building blocks of proteins). It has a pleasant flavor and leaves no bitter aftertaste. Aspartame can be used in some cooked and baked recipes but may lose its sweetness if cooked for too long or at too high temperatures. This is why it's best to add this sweetener at the end of the cooking process whenever possible. One of the amino acids in aspartame—phenylalanine—must be avoided by people who have a genetic disorder known as phenylketonuria (PKU). People who have this disorder cannot breakdown phenylalanine, so it accumulates in their blood, resulting in neurological problems. This is why aspartame-containing products are labeled with a warning to this effect.

SACCHARIN.

For many years, saccharin (sold under the brand name Sweet 'n Low) was sold with a warning that it caused cancer in laboratory animals. Recently this warning was discontinued as the FDA determined saccharine to be safe for humans to consume. Saccharine is heat stable and may be used in cooking, but used in large amounts, it has a bitter aftertaste.

SUCRALOSE.

Sold under the brand name Splenda, this sweetener is made from sucrose in a process that substitutes chlorine atoms for part of the sugar molecule. Sucralose has a natural sugar flavor, with no bitter aftertaste. It is also heat stable, so it can be used for cooking and baking. Of the products currently available on the market, sucralose is, by far, the best suited for cooking and baking.

(continued)

STEVIA.

This herbal sweetener has been used in South America for centuries. It has also been used in Japan since the early 1970s. Some brands of stevia have a slight licorice-like flavor that people might find overpowering. While stevia has no known adverse effects, it has not yet been approved by the FDA for use as a sweetener. This is why you won't find stevia sold along side other sweeteners in your grocery store. You can, however, buy stevia in health food stores, where it is sold as a dietary supplement. Realize that dietary supplements are not regulated as stringently as FDA-approved food ingredients, and may have no guarantees of purity or long-term safety.

SUGAR & OTHER CALORIC SWEETENERS.

Must you completely give up sugar to maintain a diabetes prevention lifestyle? Fortunately no. As previously mentioned, some recipes just aren't the same without a bit of real sugar. And in moderation, some sugar (and other sweeteners like honey, maple syrup, molasses, and brown sugar) *can* be included in a healthy diet—even in a diabetes prevention plan. The recipes in this book provide many examples of what we mean by moderation.

AND WHAT ABOUT "NO ADDED SUGAR"?

Just because manufacturers do not "add" sugar does not mean there's not already a whole lot of sugar in the food. Would you have thought about "no-added-sugar maple syrup?" Of course not . . . it's all sugar to begin with! So look at the label, or look up the food. The "No added . . ." label often needs to be taken with a grain of salt.

When Convenience Counts

In a perfect world, everyone would have plenty of time to prepare healthful meals from fresh ingredients every day of the week. But for most of us, this just isn't reality. What can you do when there's no time to cook? These days, most supermarkets have plenty of grab-and-go options that require little or no prep time. Here are some suggestions for putting together light and easy meals in a matter of minutes.

ENTRÉES

Most grocery stores now sell an extensive selection of heat-and-eat or ready-to-cook entrées. Some of these are very lean (3 to 5 grams of fat per serving) while others will bust your calorie budget. Here are some items that may be low in fat and calories, but always check the Nutrition Facts label to be sure.

- Precooked pot roast
- Precooked roast turkey with gravy
- Precooked roast pork loin beef tips with gravy
- Precooked corned beef or beef brisket
- Grilled chicken strips (great for making chef and Caesar salads)
- Rotisserie chicken (be sure to remove the skin)
- Marinated ready-to-cook pork tenderloins
- Marinated ready-to-cook turkey tenderloins and turkey roasts
- Ready-to-cook kebabs made with chicken or lean beef
- Precooked (steamed) shrimp

SIDES AND SALADS

- Prewashed bagged spinach. Perfect for salads or lightly sauté in a little olive oil and garlic.
- Preshredded carrots. Mix with some raisins, sliced celery, chopped apples, or canned pineapple tidbits, and a little nonfat or light mayo for a quick carrot salad.

- Baby carrots. Steam until tender and toss with a little olive oil and parsley or dill or eat raw.
- Preshredded coleslaw or broccoli slaw mix. Mix with nonfat or light mayo or coleslaw dressing for a quick and easy coleslaw. Add some diced apples, raisins, and toasted sunflower seeds for a change of pace.
- Ready-made low-fat coleslaw, tabbouleh, potato salad, and macaroni salad from your grocery deli.
- Frozen vegetable combinations.
- Ready-to-cook fresh stir-fry vegetables. Sauté with a little olive oil and toss with a low-sodium herb blend.
- Ready-to-cook collard greens and kale. Lightly sauté with a little olive oil and garlic.
- Canned sliced beets.
- Unsweetened applesauce.
- Ready-cut fresh fruit medleys.
- Microwave sweet potatoes and top with crushed pineapple or a little light margarine and a sprinkling of cinnamon (use small or halve large sweet potatoes to control carbs and calories).
- Canned reduced-fat and -sodium soups.

SOME QUICK MEAL COMBOS

Here are some tips for putting together quick and easy meals using convenience items from your grocery store.

- Rotisserie chicken (without the skin), prewashed salad mix with light vinaigrette dressing, and microwaved sweet potatoes.
- Ready-cooked lean beef roast, deli low-fat potato salad, and steamed frozen vegetable medley.
- Premarinated pork tenderloins, prewashed mixed baby salad greens with light balsamic vinaigrette dressing, boiled corn on the cob, and unsweetened applesauce.
- Ready-to-cook kebabs made with lean beef or chicken and vegetables, deli low-fat cole slaw, and ready-to-cook stir-fry vegetables sautéed in a little olive oil.

- Chef salad made with prewashed salad mix, ready-grilled chicken strips, grape tomatoes, red onion rings, shredded reduced-fat Cheddar cheese, and light ranch dressing. Pair with a cup of black bean soup.
- Spinach salad made with prewashed baby spinach topped with sliced rotisserie chicken, fresh raspberries or slivered Granny Smith apples, chopped walnuts, a sprinkling of feta cheese, and light balsamic vinaigrette dressing. Pair with a cup of lentil soup.
- Low-fat grilled cheese sandwich (coat whole-wheat bread slices very lightly with light margarine, stuff with reduced-fat cheese, and cook over medium heat in a large skillet for a couple of minutes on each side). Pair with a cup of tomato soup and some fresh-cut veggies with light ranch dip.
- Whole-wheat pita bread stuffed with ready-made hummus and salad vegetables. Pair with a cup of vegetable soup.
- Whip up an omelette or egg scramble using a fat-free egg substitute (plain or flavored with veggies or Southwestern seasonings). Fill the omelette with leftover cooked vegetables and shredded low-fat cheese. Pair with a fresh fruit cup and a toasted whole-wheat English muffin.

TIME-SAVING TIPS FOR QUICK-FIX MEALS

You've worked all day, you're tired, and you feel like you deserve a break. The last thing you want to do is whip up a full-course meal. The convenience of fast-food take-out or pizza delivery is just too much to resist. But think twice, three times, and count to ten! This scenario is all too common and can absolutely torpedo your effort to eat successfully. By using the carefully selected convenience foods discussed and applying a few other tricks, you can have an arsenal of quick *and* healthy options for home-cooked meals in a matter of minutes, and less expensively. Here are some additional strategies for success.

- Have a plan. Many people have no idea what they're having for dinner until they get home and open the refrigerator. Create a file of quick and easy recipes and meal ideas that your family enjoys for ready reference. Use these as the foundation for your menu plans.
- Make a shopping list. Plan menus a week in advance and purchase the food you need all at once. Always keep staples like canned soups, canned

tomatoes, marinara sauce, whole-wheat pasta, canned beans, tuna, and frozen veggies on hand. Stock up on the convenience items listed in the previous section.

TYPE OF RECIPE	HOW TO MAKE IT BETTER
BURGERS, MEATLOAF, MEATBALLS	Use ground meat that is at least 93% to 96% lean. Replace up to ⅓ of the ground meat with vegetarian recipe crumbles. Incorporate lots of finely chopped vegetables (mushrooms, onions, bell peppers, carrots, etc.) into the meat mixture. Substitute rolled oats or oat bran for fillers like breadcrumbs.
DEEP-FRIED FOODS	Coat the food with crushed Special-K or whole grain cereal, or toasted wheat germ. Spray lightly with cooking spray, and oven-fry instead of deep-fry.
MARINADES	Reduce the amount of sugar used. Add sweetness with fruit juices and juice concentrates instead.
SOUPS	Use lean meats and defatted stocks. Include generous amounts of vegetables and legumes in recipes. Substitute evaporated skim or low-fat milk for cream. Thicken soups with puréed vegetables instead of cream.
SALADS	Substitute lower-fat mayonnaise, sour cream, and dressings for full-fat versions. Use lower-fat meats and cheeses.
PASTA DISHES	Use lean meats, skinless chicken, and seafood in pasta dishes. Incorporate generous amounts of vegetables into pasta dishes.
QUICHES	Substitute evaporated skim or low-fat milk for cream. Substitute fat-free egg substitute for whole eggs, or use fewer yolks and more whites. Use lower-fat cheeses and lean meats.

TYPE OF RECIPE	HOW TO MAKE IT BETTER
OMELETTES, FRITTATAS	Substitute fat-free egg substitute for whole eggs, or use fewer yolks and more whites. Use lower-fat cheeses and lean meats.
CASSEROLES	Use lower-fat cheeses and sour cream. Use leaner meats. Use less butter, margarine, and oil. Substitute brown rice, wild rice, barley, or bulgur wheat for white rice.
PILAFS	Substitute brown rice, wild rice, barley, bulgur wheat, or whole-wheat couscous for white rice. Incorporate generous amounts of vegetables into the recipe.
STUFFINGS	Use whole-grain bread, brown rice, wild rice, or bulgur wheat for the stuffing base. Incorporate generous amounts of vegetables such as mushrooms, onions, carrots, and celery into the recipe.
SANDWICHES	Use hearty whole-grain bread, whole-wheat pita bread, or whole-wheat flour tortillas. Add lots of vegetable fillings. Use nonfat or light mayo or light ranch dressing instead of full-fat mayo.
FRENCH TOAST	Use whole-grain bread. Top with fresh or canned fruit, applesauce, or low-sugar fruit sauces.
PANCAKES, WAFFLES	Substitute whole-wheat flour or whole-wheat pastry flour for the white flour. Replace part of the flour with oatmeal, oat bran, or wheat germ. Top with fresh or canned fruit, applesauce, or low-sugar fruit sauces.

(continued)

TYPE OF RECIPE	HOW TO MAKE IT BETTER
MUFFINS, QUICK BREADS, COOKIES	Replace part of the white flour with whole-wheat pastry flour, oat flour, oat bran, oatmeal, flax meal, wheat bran, or wheat germ.
	Incorporate fruits, fruit juices, and dried fruits into the recipe to reduce the need for sugar.
	Add a little extra cinnamon, nutmeg, cardamom, orange rind, or vanilla extract to enhance sweetness.
	Use healthful oils like canola, soybean, and walnut.
	Substitute applesauce or puréed fruit for part of the oil.
YEAST BREADS	Use ingredients like stone-ground whole-wheat flour, oatmeal, oat bran, flax meal, wheat germ, wheat bran, nuts and seeds, soaked cracked grains, and cooked whole grains.
CUSTARDS, PUDDINGS	Substitute evaporated skim or low-fat milk for cream.
	Substitute skim or low-fat milk for whole milk. (Add a couple of tablespoons of nonfat dry milk powder per cup of milk for a richer taste.)
	Substitute fat-free egg substitutes for whole eggs.
	Add a little cinnamon, nutmeg, cardamom, orange rind, or vanilla extract to enhance sweetness.
CRISPS, COBBLERS, PIES	Prepare recipes with more fruit and less sugar.
	Use canned sugar-free or reduced-sugar pie fillings for convenience.
	Substitute oatmeal or oat bran for part of the flour in toppings and crusts.

■ Dinner does not always have to be a hot meal. There's nothing wrong with serving a hearty sandwich or chef salad for dinner.

■ Serve breakfast for dinner. Low-fat omelettes, frittatas, and whole-wheat French toast made with a fat-free egg substitute and fruit topping are great quick fixes. Round out the meal with some low-fat sausage and fresh fruit cup. There's nothing wrong with having a bowl of whole-grain cereal with nonfat milk and fruit for dinner either.

■ Plan for leftovers. Create a chef salad from leftover grilled or roasted chicken, turn leftover pot roast into hot roast beef sandwiches, use last night's brown rice in tonight's chicken casserole, or use leftover roasted asparagus in a low-fat omelette or quiche.

■ Do as much in one pot or pan as possible. Look for recipes like low-fat lasagna, beef stew, chili, and various casseroles that include several food groups and can be made in one pot or dish. Add a salad (using prewashed salad mix) or vegetable, and dinner is served!

■ Pull out the Crock Pot. Add the ingredients for a hearty bean soup, chicken and vegetables, or pot roast, and let dinner cook while you're away.

■ Make extra and freeze some for later. Soups, stews, and chili are especially good choices for freezing.

Giving Recipes a Healthy Makeover

With just a little know-how, you can easily transform your favorite family recipes into healthful and delicious, diabetes-fighting dishes. Becoming familiar with the foods described in the first part of this chapter is the first step toward healthier cooking. The table on page 86 presents some tips that will help you use these ingredients to master the basics of light and healthy cooking.

This chapter proves that eating to prevent diabetes need not mean dieting and deprivation. A wide variety of healthful and delicious foods can star in your meals, and most of these foods are readily available in your local grocery store. The later chapters of this book feature over 170 kitchen-tested recipes that put principle into practice and present a wide range of delicious possibilities for every meal for the day.

6. HAVING IT YOUR WAY IN RESTAURANTS

Nearly half of all food dollars are spent away from home. From food courts and fast food to all-you-can-eat buffets and fine dining, what we eat away from home is having a huge impact on our health, and most of it is not for the better. Restaurants want your business, and most are more than willing to let you "have it your way." The downside is that, increasingly, foods eaten away from home give supersized portions, overdosing the customer on calories, fat, and sodium.

Portion Distortion

Restaurants have led the way in supersizing food portions—and most of this food *does* end up getting eaten. One report found that a portion of fries in a fast-food chain provided 210 calories twenty years ago and 610 calories today! There is simply no question that American restaurants, compared with anywhere else in the world, give us enormous portions—and no question that our waistlines show the effect.

The more food on the plate, the more a person is likely to eat at one sitting. In fact, about two-thirds of Americans eat everything on their plate when they eat in restaurants. Not only does this cause you to feel physically uncomfortable after eating, but it often provides a huge overdose of unneeded calories.

Here are some strategies for keeping portions under control:

▩ Don't go to a restaurant ravenously hungry. Have a light snack in the afternoon to take the edge off your hunger, and you'll have more control when ordering.
▩ Request an extra plate and split an entrée with a dinner companion.
▩ Be creative. Consider ordering an à la carte meal of an appetizer, soup, and salad rather than a full-course meal.
▩ Check the menu to see if smaller or half-size entrées are offered. Some restaurants do offer these "lighter" portions at a reduced cost. If lighter portions are not available, ask if they will serve a lunch-sized portion at dinner.
▩ Request a doggie bag at the beginning of the meal and put away half your food before you begin eating.
▩ When you are comfortably full, put your napkin on your plate. This will signal your server to remove the plate from the table and prevent you from unconsciously nibbling any remaining food.

Making the Most of the Menu

Most chefs are more than happy to modify dishes to suit your nutritional preferences. Many restaurants also have websites where you can peruse menus, look up nutritional information, ask questions, and provide feedback. So don't be afraid to ask for what you want. Here are some tips for making the most of the menu in any restaurant.

COURSE	SMART EATING SUGGESTIONS
APPETIZER	Choose steamed shrimp, mussels, or oysters; tomato juice or a virgin Mary; salad with light dressing; and/or vegetable, broth-based, or bean soups.
	Skip the appetizer and save your calories for the meal.
BREAD	Most of the bread served in restaurants is made from white flour and is loaded with refined carbohydrates. Your best bet is to send back the breadbasket, or at least push it to the other side of the table.
	When ordering sandwiches, toast, and French toast, have these items made with whole-grain bread.
SALAD	Go easy on the dressing or choose a light dressing. (Just two tablespoons of full-fat dressing contains about 150 calories.) Limit toppings like cheese, bacon, and croutons.
	For extra flavor, top your salad with a tablespoon of grated Parmesan cheese (only 25 calories).
ENTRÉE	Look for menu items that are steamed, broiled, blackened, grilled, roasted, en papillote (cooked in a packet in their own juices), stir-fried, stewed, braised, or poached.
	Ask for sauces on the side.
SIDE DISHES	Substitute fresh fruit; a side salad; cup of vegetable, broth-based, or bean soup; baked sweet potato, or steamed vegetables for accompaniments like French fries, onion rings, pretzels, and chips.
	To cut back on carbs, substitute extra veggies like broccoli, green beans, or summer squash for potatoes and rice.
	Ask for extra lemon wedges to perk up vegetables and salads.
SANDWICHES	Request whole-grain bread.
	Avoid sandwiches made with overly large bagels, specialty breads, or extra-thick bread slices. Between the bread, meat, cheese, and "special sauces," supersized sandwiches can provide 700 to 1,000 calories!

COURSE	SMART EATING SUGGESTIONS
SANDWICHES (cont.)	Have sandwiches dressed with mustard, low-fat mayo, or light ranch or Italian dressing.
	Pile on plenty of lettuce, tomato, onion, peppers, sprouts, and other vegetable toppings.
BREAKFAST	Ask if you can have omelettes, scrambled eggs, and French toast made with a fat-free egg substitute or with more whites and fewer yolks.
	Request unbuttered whole-wheat toast instead of buttered white toast.
	Have French toast made with whole-wheat bread.
	Order Canadian bacon instead of regular bacon or sausage.
	Look for menu items like oatmeal, yogurt, and fruit.
	Ask for milk for your coffee or tea instead of cream.
DESSERT	If you want dessert, share it with a friend—or with several friends. Remember, you get the most pleasure from the first couple of bites.
	Be aware that the "low-fat" and "sugar-free" desserts featured at some restaurants can still be loaded with calories. This is because sugar-free desserts can be full of fat while fat-free desserts may be excessively high in sugar.

Getting Down to Specifics

Each type of restaurant poses its challenges and rewards, but with just a little insight and creativity, you can easily enjoy a healthful and delicious meal at just about any restaurant. Here are some tips for making the most of your dining experience in a variety of different settings.

CHINESE	
FOODS TO CHOOSE	**FOODS TO AVOID**
Broth-based soups like wonton, hot and sour, and egg drop; steamed dumplings	Fried egg rolls, fried wontons, fried noodles, spare ribs, chicken wings
Stir-fried combinations of seafood, poultry, lean meat, tofu, and vegetables (ask for less oil than usual to be used in preparation)	Stir-fried dishes that contain battered and deep-fried meats (like sweet and sour pork dishes)
Steamed fish and vegetable dishes	Dishes made with duck (duck is very fatty)
Chop suey, chow mein (served plain or with a moderate portion of rice or nonfried noodles instead of fried chow mein noodles)	Egg foo yung
	Crispy fish and crispy chicken (these dishes are fried)
Stir-fried noodle dishes like seafood, chicken, or vegetable lo mein (ask for less oil than usual to be used in preparation)	Fried rice
Steamed brown rice (if available)	Use sweet sauces, such as sweet & sour, hoisin, and plum, in limited amounts.
Szechuan sauce, bean sauce, shrimp sauce, oyster sauce, hot mustard	
Fortune cookie (one fortune cookie has only 30 calories and 6 grams of carbohydrate)	

FRENCH	
FOODS TO CHOOSE	**FOODS TO AVOID**
Consommé and broth-based soups, steamed mussels	Vichyssoise (creamy potato soup) and other cream soups, pâté (liver, meat, or chicken spreads made with cream, butter, and egg yolks)
Broiled, steamed, or poached seafood and poultry (order sauces on the side)	

FRENCH *(cont.)*	
FOODS TO CHOOSE	FOODS TO AVOID
Seafood and poultry cooked en papillote (steamed in parchment paper)	High-fat sauces like Hollandaise and béarnaise (made with egg yolks and butter, these sauces contain about 200 calories and 20 fat grams per ¼ cup)
Chicken or fish Provençal (with tomato sauce), chicken or fish cooked with tomato-wine sauces	Remoulade sauce (a mayonnaise-based sauce typically served with seafood)
Seafood or vegetable stews such as bouillabaisse and ratatouille	Quiches, soufflés, and crêpes (these dishes are typically made with unhealthy amounts of cream, cheese, butter, and egg yolks)
Chicken and beef stews with wine or tomato sauces	Croissants (high in refined carbs and fat)
Steamed vegetables, salads with dressing on the side	French bread (limit portions—high in refined carbs)
Sherbets, sorbets, poached fruits, fresh fruits with liqueur	Crème fraîche (thickened, cultured heavy cream)
	Brie, Camembert, Roquefort, Boursin, and other fatty cheeses
	French pastries, cakes, cheesecake, mousse, crème brûlée, and other high-fat desserts

GREEK	
FOODS TO CHOOSE	FOODS TO AVOID
Bean and lentil soups, avgolemono (lemon and egg) soup, vegetable soups, fish soups	Buttery, phyllo-crusted dishes such as spanokopita (spinach pie)
Souvlaki (shish kebabs) of chicken, lean beef or pork, roasted lamb, and vegetables	Dolmades (grape leaves stuffed with high-fat ground meat and rice)

(continued)

GREEK	
FOODS TO CHOOSE	**FOODS TO AVOID**
Baked fish dishes such as plaki (fish baked with tomatoes, onions, and garlic) and fish baked in grape leaves; baked chicken dishes (ask the chef to use a minimal amount of butter or oil in baked dishes)	Dishes loaded with creamy or cheesy sauces like moussaka (ground meat and eggplant casserole)
Gyro sandwiches made with grilled chicken	Baklava (phyllo pastry made with butter, nuts, and honey), nut cakes, butter cookies
Greek salads made with a light sprinkling of feta cheese and vinaigrette dressing on the side	
Fruit compotes, marinated fruits	

INDIAN	
FOODS TO CHOOSE	**FOODS TO AVOID**
Vegetable and dal (lentil or bean) soups	Coconut soup
Vegetable, seafood, and chicken curry dishes (except for those made with large amounts of coconut or coconut milk)	Samosa (fried turnovers), pakora (fried chicken or vegetable fritters), and papadum (crisp fried lentil wafers)
Chicken or shrimp vindaloo (in a hot and spicy tomato, onion, and curry sauce)	Dishes made with coconut milk or cream
Tandoori chicken or fish (chicken marinated in yogurt and spices and baked in a clay oven)	Dishes made with large amounts of ghee (clarified butter)
Lamb or chicken kabobs	Puri (fried bread)
Chapati (a whole-wheat tortillalike bread), roti and naan (oven-baked flatbreads)	
Vegetable, chicken, or seafood biryanis (rice-based dishes)	

INDIAN *(cont.)*	
FOODS TO CHOOSE	**FOODS TO AVOID**
Raita (a cold side dish made of cucumbers or other vegetables with yogurt sauce) Chutney (a spicy accompaniment to meals)	

ITALIAN	
FOODS TO CHOOSE	**FOODS TO AVOID**
Vegetable or bean-based soups like minestrone and pasta fagioli	Meat and cheese antipasto platters
Steamed clams or mussels	Fried calamari and fried mozzarella
Moderate portions of pasta with tomato-based sauces (like marinara, puttanesca, and arrabbiata); pasta with tomato-seafood sauces like red clam sauce	Pasta with creamy sauces like alfredo and carbonara
Broiled or grilled chicken and fish dishes	Cheese-laden dishes like lasagna, cheese manicotti, and cannelloni
Chicken cacciatore; chicken or veal picatta and marsala (request that only a small amount of fat be used to prepare these dishes)	Dishes like eggplant and veal parmigiana that are battered, fried, and covered with cheese Dishes made with Italian sausage
Seafood stews like cioppino	Pizza with extra cheese, olive oil, and meat toppings
Thin crust pizza with vegetable toppings	Italian bread, focaccia, and breadsticks (limit amounts—high in refined carbohydrates)
Granita, poached fruits, biscotti, amaretti cookies, cappuccino made with low-fat milk	Cheesecake, tiramisu, Italian pastries and cookies, spumoni, mousse

(continued)

JAPANESE	
FOODS TO CHOOSE	**FOODS TO AVOID**
Miso soup, broth-based soup	Fried dumplings
Steamed dumplings	Sushi made with fried fish, mayonnaise, cream cheese, or other high-fat ingredients
Sushi (vinegared rice, raw fish, and/or vegetables rolled or pressed together into small morsels), sashimi (raw, slivered fish, usually served with a dipping sauce)	Tempura (batter-coated and fried foods)
	Tonkatsu (deep-fried pork), torikatsu (deep-fried chicken), katsudon (deep-fried pork, onion, and egg)
Yakitori (broiled chicken kebabs), teriyaki dishes, "yakimono" (grilled) dishes, sukiyaki (thinly sliced beef and vegetables in a piquant, slightly sweet sauce), wasabi (Japanese horseradish)	Fried rice
Stir-fried seafood, chicken, lean beef, or tofu and vegetable combinations	
Udon (wheat) noodles, soba (buckwheat) noodles, rice noodles, steamed brown rice (if available)	
MEXICAN	
FOODS TO CHOOSE	**FOODS TO AVOID**
Black bean soup, seviche (lime-marinated seafood salad), gazpacho (chilled tomato and cucumber soup)	Fried tortilla chips, nachos
	Sour cream, cheese
Grilled fish and chicken dishes	Fried entrées like chimichangas and chili rellenos
	Enchiladas (the tortillas are typically softened by drenching in oil)

MEXICAN *(cont.)*	
FOODS TO CHOOSE	FOODS TO AVOID
Chicken soft tacos and *small* burritos. Note: when choosing tortilla-based entrées, avoid those made with supersize tortilla wraps and rice fillings, as they can easily provide a carbohydrate overdose. Also, see if whole wheat tortillas are available and limit the high-fat cheese and sour cream. Salsa, tomatillo sauce, verde (green) sauce, pico de gallo (tomatoes with onions and hot peppers) Guacamole (healthy but high in calories)	Refried beans and Mexican rice side dishes (both usually contain an unhealthy amount of lard or other fat)

THAI	
FOODS TO CHOOSE	FOODS TO AVOID
Broth-based soups like Tom Yum Gai (chicken with vegetables and Thai seasonings) or Tom Yum Goong (shrimp with vegetables and Thai seasonings), and steamed dumplings Stir-fried combinations of seafood, chicken, tofu, lean meat, and vegetables (ask for less oil than usual to be used in preparation) Moderate portions of Pad-thai and other stir-fried noodle dishes made with vegetables and seafood, chicken, tofu, or lean meat (ask for less oil than usual to be used in preparation) Dishes made with basil sauce, lime sauce, chili sauce, and fish sauce	Coconut soup, chicken wings, egg rolls, wontons, and other fried appetizers Dishes made with duck (duck is very fatty) Deep-fried dishes like crispy noodles and crispy fish Fried rice dishes Fried noodles Dishes made with coconut milk

(continued)

STEAK HOUSES	
FOODS TO CHOOSE	FOODS TO AVOID
Shish kebabs	Greasy appetizers like deep-fried whole onions, cheese fries
Small sirloin or tenderloin (filet mignon) steaks	Fatty meats like New York strip, T-bone, porterhouse, rib eye, prime rib, pork chops
Grilled or barbecued skinless chicken, grilled fish	Baked potatoes loaded with butter and sour cream, French fries
Grilled steak or chicken salads with light dressing (limit cheese and bacon toppings)	The bread basket
Side salad with light dressing, steamed or grilled vegetables, baked sweet potatoes	

PIZZERIAS	
FOODS TO CHOOSE	FOODS TO AVOID
Thin crust pizza	Thick crust, stuffed crust, double-crust pizzas
Part-skim mozzarella cheese (if available)	Whole-milk cheese (if whole milk cheese is all that's available, ask for half the cheese, or just have your pizza topped with a sprinkling of grated Parmesan cheese instead of mozzarella)
Vegetable toppings—onions, green bell peppers, mushrooms, sun-dried tomatoes, artichoke hearts, roasted red bell peppers, broccoli, spinach, zucchini, etc.	
Roasted chicken, ham, or Canadian bacon toppings	High-fat meat toppings like sausage, pepperoni, and ground beef
Side salad	Extras like breadsticks and cheese bread (there's enough carbohydrate in the crust)

FAST FOOD	
FOODS TO CHOOSE	**FOODS TO AVOID**
Grilled chicken sandwiches, pitas, or wraps (spread with mustard, light mayo, light ranch, or light Italian dressing); plain small burgers, roast beef sandwiches	Supersize burgers
	Fried chicken or fish sandwiches
	Sandwiches made with extra-thick or supersize bread
Light six-inch subs on whole-grain bread with plenty of vegetable toppings (like Subway)	
Grilled chicken salads with light dressing, side salads with light dressing, taco salads (omit the fried shell or tortilla chips and limit the sour cream and cheese toppings), Caesar salads (use only half the dressing or substitute light Italian dressing)	Taco salads served in fried shells; Caesar salads tossed in oily dressings (these salads can have as much as 700 calories and over 40 grams of fat)
	Supersize fries
Chili, bean burritos, chicken fajitas	High-fat milk shakes, sundaes, cookies, fried apple pies, and other high-calorie desserts
Thin crust pizza with vegetable toppings, lean ham, or Canadian bacon (Add a side salad for nutritional balance)	Thick crust or stuffed crust pizzas with extra cheese and meat toppings
Frozen yogurt, low-fat ice cream/ice milk	

As you have seen, adopting a diabetes prevention lifestyle does not have to mean giving up the pleasures of dining out. From fast-food to fine dining, many excellent choices are available. The restaurant industry has become very aware that people want better choices, and most establishments are more than happy to accommodate special dietary requests. Many restaurants are also offering lighter fare that fits perfectly with your diabetes prevention plan. By using the tips provided in this chapter, you can enjoy a healthful and delicious meal at just about any restaurant.

7. THE POWER OF PHYSICAL ACTIVITY

Everyone can benefit from exercise, but people who are at risk for diabetes probably have the most to gain from being active. There is no question that an active lifestyle can combat insulin resistance and prevent or delay type 2 diabetes. But how much exercise is enough—and which type is best? This chapter answers these questions and provides simple, doable strategies that prove that exercise need not be grueling, complicated, or overly time-consuming to be highly effective.

How Physical Activity Fights Diabetes

Many of the health benefits of exercise are immediate and occur even if you don't lose weight. This is especially true for the exercise-induced changes that fight diabetes. What happens when you adopt an active lifestyle?

- Exercise acts much like an "insulin-sensitizing" drug to make the body's cells more responsive to insulin and enable them to remove glucose from the blood more efficiently. As a result, the pancreas does not have to secrete as much insulin to keep blood sugar under control. Reducing the workload of the pancreas helps preserve its ability to function.

■ Exercise helps lower blood sugar by directly burning glucose for fuel.

■ Exercise helps you lose body fat (especially abdominal fat), which also lowers diabetes risk.

In addition to reducing diabetes risk, exercise can enhance your life in many other ways. Most people report an immediate increase in energy level and quickly develop better muscular strength and endurance. Their mood improves and they feel less stressed. Within weeks, muscles start to appear more toned and their clothes fit more loosely.

Exercise also dramatically lowers your risk for cardiovascular disease, the number-one killer of people with diabetes. How? Regular exercise increases HDL ("good") cholesterol and lowers blood triglycerides. It can also help reduce blood pressure and decrease clotting in the blood. The heart muscle becomes stronger and blood flows more efficiently throughout the body.

Rounding out this list of added benefits, exercise builds stronger bones and reduces the risk of osteoporosis. It also lowers the risk of some cancers. Exercise has been found to improve memory and slow the age-related decline in mental function. It can improve sexual functioning and makes people feel better about their bodies.

TELEVISION WATCHING AND DIABETES RISK

Researchers have long known that a couch-potato lifestyle sets the stage for diabetes. This is because sedentary muscles lose their ability to respond to insulin, which leads to higher blood insulin levels and eventually higher blood sugar levels. A recent study from Harvard University found that men who spent the most time watching television (forty hours/week) nearly tripled their risk of diabetes compared to men who rarely watched television. Simply substituting physical activity for watching television or sitting at the computer could go a long way toward reducing diabetes risk. Alternatively, make the most of your TV time by using your treadmill, stationary bike, hand weights, or engaging in other physical activities while watching your favorite shows.

The bottom line is, exercise can provide big benefits for your diabetes prevention program and your overall health and wellness. The sooner you get started the better!

Getting Started

It's never too late to begin a fitness program—even if you have never exercised before. The kinds of activities that reduce diabetes risk and improve overall health do not require a high level of athletic skill. Here are some tips for getting started:

CONSULT YOUR PHYSICIAN

If you have been sedentary for a while, are over age forty-five, significantly overweight, or are being treated for medical conditions such as heart disease, high blood pressure, prediabetes, or diabetes, you should consult with a physician before embarking on an exercise program. This will give you a chance to have your blood pressure, cholesterol, and blood sugar levels checked. Your doctor may have specific recommendations for exercising based on any physical limitations that you might have.

SET REALISTIC GOALS

If you can realistically commit to only thirty minutes three times a week, then make that your initial goal. People who overdo it set themselves up for frustration, injury, and burnout. It's much better to start slowly and gradually increase your program. Set small, short-term goals such as walking around the block without becoming winded. Next, expand your walk to two blocks, and then pick up the pace a little to cover more territory in the same span of time.

FIND A PARTNER

When you have an exercise buddy, physical activity becomes more of a fun, social event. You are more likely to continue with your program if you have a commitment to be there for your partner and they commit to being there for you.

REWARD YOURSELF FOR A JOB WELL DONE

A good way to maintain motivation is to reward yourself for accomplishing a goal. For instance, if you meet your monthly exercise goal, reward yourself with a new workout outfit, an evening at the theater, or other incentives. Just avoid using food as a reward!

How Much Is Enough?

Many health benefits can be derived from just adding thirty minutes of moderate-intensity exercise to your daily life. However, this is not enough to prevent the "creeping weight gain syndrome" in most people. So for optimal health and better weight control, the National Academy of Sciences Institute of Medicine recommends accumulating an hour of physical activity daily.

If you're wondering where you will find the time to do this, you will be relieved to know that your hour of physical activity can be done all at once or divided into several smaller bouts, giving you plenty of flexibility. Everyday activities like housework, yard work, washing the car, and walking the dog can all count, so this is definitely doable. The important thing is to just get moving.

It's crucial that you choose enjoyable activities so that your exercise program does not become just another chore. For instance, socialize with a friend over a walk, bike ride, or canoe trip instead of watching television or going out to eat. Plant a vegetable or flower garden, walk the dog, or take a family hike. Take the stairs instead of the elevator. Walk to lunch. It all adds up.

SOME WAYS TO ADD EXERCISE TO YOUR LIFE

- Make exercise a social event—meet up with a friend at the gym, for a walk, or for a game of tennis.
- Take a short walk on your work breaks.
- Take the stairs instead of the elevator or escalator.
- Park farther away when you go shopping and run errands. Or get off the subway or bus a stop earlier and walk to your destination.
- Enjoy walks with your dog.

CALORIES BURNED DURING SELECTED ACTIVITIES

Exercise is a must for losing weight and keeping it off. Indeed, studies show that people who are successful at long-term weight loss burn about 400 calories per day with exercise. Increasing your activity level to burn just 100 extra calories a day can produce a ten-pound weight loss over the course of a year!

ACTIVITY	CALORIES BURNED PER 30 MINUTES*
Basketball	282
Canoeing (leisure)	90
Circuit training	218
Cleaning	120
Cycling (9.4 mph)	204
Dancing (ballroom)	105
Mowing yard (push mower)	228
Racquetball	363
Running (9-minute miles)	393
Scrubbing floors	222
Swimming (fast crawl)	318
Tennis	222
Volleyball	102
Walking	162
Window cleaning	120

*Based on a 150-pound person. Smaller and larger people will burn proportionately fewer or more calories.

- View household chores like cleaning, raking leaves, mowing the yard, shoveling snow, chopping firewood, and washing the car as opportunities to be more active.
- Plan a hike or biking excursion with family or friends.
- Exercise while watching television.
- Join an aerobics, body shaping, Pilates, yoga, or other fitness class.
- Plant a vegetable, herb, or flower garden.
- Wear a pedometer to track the number of steps you take in a day. Two-thousand steps is the equivalent of one mile.
- Instead of lying around the pool, jump in and do some laps or pool exercises.

Which Kind of Exercise Is Best?

The truth is any kind of exercise can help reduce diabetes risk—so if you are currently sedentary, just pick something and start moving. Most people find walking to be the simplest and most enjoyable way to add exercise to their life. However, two main categories of exercise offer unique health benefits for diabetes prevention and for overall health. A well-rounded exercise program includes some of each type. The exercise pyramid on page 110 puts these into perspective.

AEROBIC EXERCISE

Aerobic exercise encompasses a wide variety of low- to moderate-intensity activities such as walking, jogging, biking, racquet sports, swimming, and dancing. Activities like raking leaves, using a push mower, and mopping the floor can also be considered aerobic exercise. These forms of exercise are fueled mostly by fat, which can be burned only when there is an adequate supply of oxygen present in the exercising muscles.

Aerobic exercise requires the body to use increased amounts of oxygen, which makes the heart and lungs work harder. When you engage in this kind of exercise regularly, your cardiovascular system becomes stronger and more efficient at delivering oxygen throughout the body. Some specific benefits that occur with aerobic exercise include:

- Your heart becomes larger and stronger and pumps more blood with each beat. As a result, your pulse rate slows.

- Blood pressure falls as blood flows more easily through your veins and arteries.
- Blood cholesterol and triglycerides levels drop and HDL ("good") cholesterol rises.
- Your lungs gain strength and endurance, so breathing becomes more efficient.
- The exercising muscles become more toned.
- Muscles develop more fat-burning enzymes and become more efficient at burning fat both during exercise and at rest.
- Muscles become more sensitive to insulin, which helps keep blood sugar levels under control and reduces the risk for diabetes.
- Your immune system becomes stronger, reducing your risk for all kinds of illnesses.

Try to accumulate thirty to sixty minutes of aerobic exercise throughout the day. This can be done all at once or in several bouts of at least ten-minutes each.

PICK UP THE PACE

When it comes to walking, brisk is better. One study found that women who described their walking pace as "brisk" were more than 40 percent less likely to develop type 2 diabetes as were women who described their pace as "easy, casual." What's considered brisk? If you can walk a mile in fifteen minutes (four miles per hour), you're doing a brisk walk.

STRENGTH TRAINING

Strength training (also called resistance training) is any exercise that makes muscles work against some kind of resistance, such as weight lifting, calisthenics (like push-ups and pull-ups), and body-shaping classes that use free weights or resistance tubes. Activities like chopping and stacking firewood, gardening and heavy yard work (digging, hoeing, pushing a wheelbarrow, etc.), and chores like shoveling snow also build muscles.

Strength training has emerged as a powerful diabetes prevention strategy in recent years. The reason? As people get older, diabetes risk rises partly because of the loss of muscle mass that occurs. Muscle is the body's main "clearinghouse" for blood glucose, accounting for about 75 percent of glucose disposal by the body. Maintaining a healthy proportion of lean body mass is key to keeping blood sugar levels under control—and strength training is the most effective type of exercise for building and maintaining muscle.

Most people can reap additional benefits by supplementing their aerobic activities with strength training. Here are some examples:

■ As you build muscle mass, your metabolic rate increases, causing you to burn more calories and making it easier to lose body fat.

■ Your body becomes firmer and denser. You may notice that your clothes fit looser even if you don't lose weight. This happens because muscle weighs more than fat. If your primary goal is weight loss, don't be discouraged if you don't lose weight as quickly as you would like. Let your appearance be your guide and monitor your results by tracking changes in body measurements or percentage of body fat.

■ Muscles become more sensitive to insulin, which helps to keep blood sugar levels under control and reduces the risk of diabetes.

■ Bones become stronger and denser and less likely to fracture. Your risk of osteoporosis declines.

■ Building stronger muscles helps prevent falls, improve mobility, and counteract frailty that occurs with aging.

We could spend a lot of time prescribing a detailed strength-training program with specific exercise sequences and go on and on about the optimal number of repetitions and sets—but the truth is it doesn't have to be that complicated. A total body strength-training regimen can be accomplished with as little as two one-hour sessions per week. You can strength-train in a gym or in the privacy of your own home using an instructional videotape and hand weights or other equipment. A basic program includes eight to ten different exercises that work the muscles of the legs, trunk, arms, chest, and shoulders. However, many people choose to train more intensely and more often for larger strength gains and improved muscle tone. Remember, too, that if you regularly engage in vigorous activities like gardening, shoveling, digging, etc. you may not need any additional strength training.

CUT DOWN ON

WATCHING TELEVISION, COMPUTER TIME

2–3 TIMES A WEEK

WEIGHT TRAINING, BODY SHAPING CLASSES
WITH WEIGHTS, HEAVY YARD WORK, ETC.

3–5 TIMES A WEEK

BRISK WALKING OR JOGGING, BIKING, SKATING,
SWIMMING; SPORTS SUCH AS TENNIS, SOFTBALL
RACQUETBALL, BASKETBALL, ETC.

DO DAILY

PARK FARTHER AWAY, TAKE THE STAIRS, WALK THE DOG,
WORK IN YOUR GARDEN, HOUSEWORK, ETC.

Exercise Pyramid for a Well-Rounded Program of Physical Activity

A Word about Stretching

Remaining flexible is key to maintaining balance and agility throughout life. Being flexible also helps prevent injuries during exercise and everyday activities. You can improve flexibility by stretching at home and/or participating in activities such as yoga, Pilates, and tai chi. Stretch all the major muscle groups at least twice a week and include stretches as part of your warm-up and cooldown before and after exercise.

Use It or Lose It

The health benefits of exercise start to subside once you stop an exercise program and are completely lost within a week or two. This is why it's so important to exercise *regularly*. Numerous studies show that exercise can be just as effective—or even more effective—

WHAT YOU SHOULD KNOW ABOUT HIRING A PERSONAL TRAINER

Starting a fitness program can be a daunting task, so many people hire a personal trainer. In your quest for quality, you make sure to find a "certified" personal trainer. But does that mean your trainer is qualified? Not always. Most states do not regulate personal trainers so that "certification" could mean that he or she only attended a weekend seminar or took a course over the Internet. Here are some tips for finding a qualified trainer:

- Inquire about the background of a trainer. Do they have a degree in a health-related field? How much experience do they have? Are they qualified to work with people who have medical conditions?
- Choose a gym that imposes strict standards on trainers. Some gyms require trainers to have a degree in a health-related field and/or pass a respected certification exam like that of the American College of Sports Medicine.
- Beware of trainers who push too hard, set unrealistic goals, or recommend supplements or diet programs. Most trainers have no formal training in nutrition and there have been many cases of trainers causing harm by recommending dangerous supplements and diets. Bad advice can be especially detrimental for people with medical problems such as high blood pressure, metabolic syndrome, prediabetes, diabetes, and heart disease.
- Beware of trainers who are trying to sell you something—find out if they are getting a commission.

than medications for preventing or treating prediabetes, insulin resistance, and the metabolic syndrome. Like a prescription medication, physical activity is most effective when you get your daily dose. Unlike medication though, physical activity does not have to cost anything or have negative side effects.

In summary, physical activity is every bit as important to your diabetes prevention program as eating well. Any amount of physical activity is better than none at all, and many health benefits can be derived from being active for just thirty minutes daily. Ideally, people should strive to accumulate an hour of physical activity into their daily lives, as this amount provides additional benefits and is more effective at fostering a healthy body weight. A well-rounded fitness program includes aerobic activities, strength training, and stretching exercises. Routine activities like gardening, housework, washing the car, and walking the dog can all contribute toward your daily activity goal.

There's no question that people who live an active lifestyle are a lot less likely to develop diabetes. By choosing a variety of activities that you truly enjoy, you can achieve long-term success with your fitness program. The sooner you get moving the better. Your only side effects will be more energy, a healthier body composition, and improved overall health!

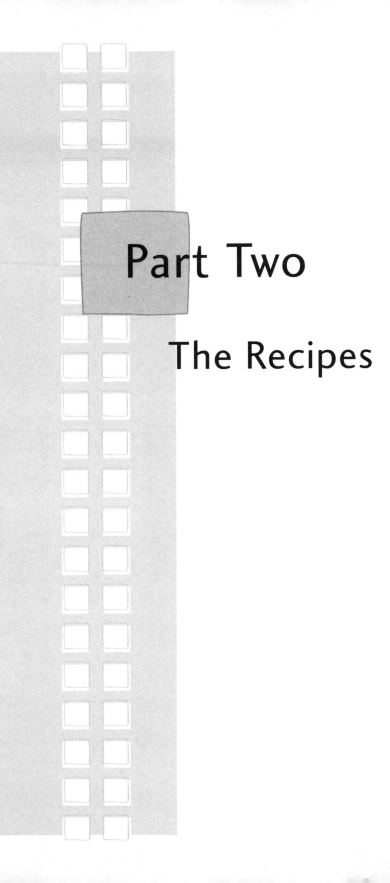

Part Two

The Recipes

About the Nutrition Analysis

As these recipes were developed, every effort was made to keep calories under control. Carbs are kept at low to moderate levels, and fats are used moderately with a focus on "good" fats. This allows you to enjoy generous and filling portions of healthful and tasty dishes without blowing your calorie budget and without sacrificing your future health.

The Food Processor nutrition analysis software (ESHA Research), along with product information from manufacturers, was used to calculate the nutrition information for the recipes in this book. For each recipe, information on calories, carbohydrate, dietary fiber, protein, fat, saturated fat, cholesterol, sodium, and calcium is provided. The serving size or unit upon which the nutrition analysis is based is clearly indicated for each recipe.

In addition to the nutrition analysis, diabetic exchanges are provided for each recipe to assist people who use this meal-planning technique. The Exchange Lists are a meal-planning system that is sometimes used for devising diabetic and weight-loss diets. Foods that are similar in carbohydrate, protein, and fat content are grouped together into an "exchange list." Thus, any food on a list can be substituted or exchanged for another. More information on using exchanges is available through your registered dietitian or diabetes educator. For all recipes except desserts, diabetic exchanges are broken down in-to meat, milk, vegetable, starch, fruit, and fat servings. Dessert recipes are broken down into more general "carbohydrate" exchanges so you can easily exchange them for other carbo-hydrate equivalents such as starches, fruit, and milk in your diet.

Sometimes recipes give options regarding ingredients. For instance, you might be able to choose between nonfat and reduced-fat cheese, eggs or egg substitute, sugar substitute or sugar, or margarine or butter. This will help you create dishes that suit your tastes and your nutrition goals. Just bear in mind that the nutrition analysis is based on the first in-gredient listed and does not include optional ingredients.

8. BREAKFAST AND BRUNCH FAVORITES

What and *when* you eat are key components of your diabetes prevention program. Breakfast is a case in point. Besides packing in fiber and essential nutrients, eating a healthy breakfast can help prevent overeating later in the day.

Beware though; all breakfast foods are not created equal. Selections like white bagels, cereal bars, toaster pastries, and many breakfast cereals are high in refined carbs and low in fiber and protein. These foods can wreak havoc on your blood sugar, trigger hunger, and lead to a pattern of overeating all day long.

This chapter will get your day off to a great start with a variety of breakfast favorites made the light and healthy way. The fiber-rich grains and lean-protein foods in these recipes will get you going and keep you feeling full and satisfied all morning long.

Looking for a change of pace at dinner? Think breakfast. A frittata or omelette served with a slice of hearty whole-grain toast and a bowl of fresh fruit makes for a quick and satisfying meal. By the same token, don't limit yourself to just breakfast foods at breakfast. There's nothing wrong with having some low-fat chicken salad with a wedge of melon, a turkey sandwich on whole wheat, or even last night's leftovers for breakfast.

Ham & Asparagus Omelette

YIELD: 1 SERVING

⅓ cup 1-inch pieces fresh asparagus

3 tablespoons diced, lean, reduced-sodium ham

½ cup fat-free egg substitute

3 tablespoons shredded nonfat or reduced-fat
   white cheddar, Monterey Jack, or Swiss
   cheese

1 tablespoon chopped, seeded plum tomato

1. Coat an 8-inch nonstick skillet with nonstick cooking spray and preheat over medium heat. Add the asparagus and ham, cover, and cook for about 3 minutes, stirring a couple of times, until the asparagus is crisp-tender and the ham is beginning to brown. Remove the asparagus and ham to a small dish and cover to keep warm.

2. Respray the skillet and place over medium-low heat. Add the egg substitute and cook without stirring for 2 minutes, until set around the edges.

3. Use a spatula to lift the edges of the omelette, and allow the uncooked egg to flow below the cooked portion. Cook for another minute or two, or until the eggs are almost set.

4. Arrange the asparagus and ham and then the cheese over half of the omelette. Fold the other half over the filling and cook for another minute or two, until the cheese is melted and the eggs are completely set.

5. Slide the omelette onto a plate, top with the chopped tomato, and serve hot.

Nutritional Facts (per serving)

CALORIES: 123 CARBOHYDRATES: 7 g
CHOLESTEROL: 14 mg FAT: 1 g SAT. FAT: 0.3 g
FIBER: 0.8 g PROTEIN: 22 g SODIUM: 619 mg
CALCIUM: 189 mg
   Diabetic exchanges: 3 very lean meat, 1 vegetable

▪ ▪ ▪

Portabella Mushroom Omelette

YIELD: 1 SERVING

Olive oil cooking spray

4 slices (¼-inch thick) portabella mushroom

¼ teaspoon herb blend (like Mrs. Dash with
   tomato, basil, and garlic)

Pinch ground black pepper

½ cup fat-free egg substitute

3 tablespoons nonfat or reduced-fat mozzarella,
   Swiss, or provolone cheese

½ teaspoon dried parsley

1. Coat an 8-inch nonstick skillet with the cooking spray and preheat over medium-high heat. Add the mushrooms and sprinkle with the herb blend and pepper. Cook for about 1 minute, until nicely browned on the bottoms. Spray the mushrooms with the cooking spray, turn, and cook for another minute, until the mushrooms are tender. Remove the

mushrooms to a small dish and cover to keep warm.

2. Respray the skillet and place over medium-low heat. Add the egg substitute and cook without stirring for 2 minutes, until set around the edges.

3. Use a spatula to lift the edges of the omelette, and allow the uncooked egg to flow below the cooked portion. Cook for another minute or two, until the eggs are almost set.

4. Arrange the mushrooms and then the cheese over half of the omelette. Fold the other half over the filling and cook for another minute or two, until the cheese is melted and the eggs are completely set.

5. Slide the omelette onto a plate, finely crumble the parsley over the top, and serve hot.

Nutritional Facts (per serving)

CALORIES: 91 CARBOHYDRATES: 4 g CHOLESTEROL: 2 mg FAT: 0.3 g SAT. FAT: 0 g FIBER: 0.3 g PROTEIN: 17 g SODIUM: 427 mg CALCIUM: 185 mg

Diabetic exchanges: 3 very lean meat, ½ vegetable

▨ ▨ ▨

Primavera Omelette

YIELD: 1 SERVING

2 tablespoons chopped onion

2 tablespoons chopped red bell pepper

¼ cup sliced mushrooms

⅛ teaspoon dried oregano

⅓ cup (packed) chopped fresh spinach

½ cup fat-free egg substitute

2 teaspoons grated Parmesan cheese

¼ teaspoon dried parsley, finely crumbled

1. Coat an 8-inch nonstick skillet with nonstick cooking spray and preheat over medium heat. Add onion, bell pepper, mushrooms, and oregano. Cover, and cook for about 2 minutes, stirring a couple of times, until the vegetables are tender. Add the spinach and cook for another minute, until the spinach is wilted. Remove the vegetable mixture to a small dish and cover to keep warm.

2. Respray the skillet and place over medium-low heat. Add the egg substitute and cook without stirring for 2 minutes, until set around the edges.

3. Use a spatula to lift the edges of the omelette, and allow the uncooked egg to flow below the cooked portion. Cook for another minute or two, until the eggs are almost set.

4. Arrange the vegetable mixture over half of the omelette and sprinkle with the cheese. Fold the other half over the filling and cook for another minute or two, until the eggs are completely set.

5. Slide the omelette onto a plate, top with the parsley, and serve hot.

Nutritional Facts (per serving)

CALORIES: 96 CARBOHYDRATES: 6 g CHOLESTEROL: 3 mg FAT: 1.4 g SAT. FAT: 0.8 g FIBER: 1 g PROTEIN: 15 g SODIUM: 337 mg CALCIUM: 113 mg

Diabetic exchanges: 2 very lean meat, 1 vegetable

▨ ▨ ▨

Omelette with Sun-Dried Tomatoes, Mushrooms, & Onions

YIELD: 1 SERVING

⅓ cup sliced fresh mushrooms

2 thin slices yellow onion

2 to 3 teaspoons sun-dried tomatoes packed in olive oil, drained

1 teaspoon prepared pesto

½ cup fat-free egg substitute

1 tablespoon shredded Parmesan cheese

½ teaspoon dried parsley

1. Coat an 8-inch nonstick skillet with nonstick cooking spray and preheat over medium heat. Add the mushrooms and onion. Cover and cook for about 2 minutes, stirring a couple of times, until the vegetables are tender. Remove the vegetable mixture to a small dish, stir in the tomatoes and pesto, and cover to keep warm.

2. Respray the skillet and place over medium-low heat. Add the egg substitute and cook without stirring for 2 minutes, until set around the edges.

3. Use a spatula to lift the edges of the omelette and allow the uncooked egg to flow below the cooked portion. Cook for another minute or two, until the eggs are almost set.

4. Arrange the vegetable mixture over half of the omelette and sprinkle with the Parme-san cheese. Fold the other half over the filling and cook for another minute or two, until the eggs are completely set.

5. Slide the omelette onto a plate, finely crumble the parsley over the top, and serve hot.

Nutritional Facts (per serving)

CALORIES: 137 CARBOHYDRATES: 8 g
CHOLESTEROL: 5 mg FAT: 4.5 g SAT. FAT: 1.6 g
FIBER: 1.5 g PROTEIN: 16 g SODIUM: 389 mg
CALCIUM: 152 mg

Diabetic exchanges: 2 lean meat, 1 vegetable

Zucchini-Onion Frittata

YIELD: 4 SERVINGS

2 cups fat-free egg substitute

¼ cup grated Parmesan cheese

1 tablespoon extra virgin olive oil

2 medium zucchini squashes, thinly sliced

1 medium yellow onion, thinly sliced

1 teaspoon crushed garlic

¼ teaspoon salt

¼ teaspoon ground black pepper

1. Preheat the oven to 350 degrees. In a medium bowl, whisk together the eggs and Parmesan cheese and set aside.

2. Coat the bottom and sides of a large, nonstick, oven-proof skillet with cooking spray and add the olive oil. Add the zucchini, onions, garlic, salt, and pepper and sauté over

medium-high heat for several minutes, until tender. Spread the mixture evenly over the bottom of the skillet.

3. Pour the egg mixture over the vegetables. Cook without stirring for 3 minutes, until the bottom of the frittata is just set.

4. Place the frittata in the oven and bake uncovered for 12 to 15 minutes or until the eggs are set but not dry. Loosen the edges of the frittata and invert it onto a plate. Cut the frittata into 4 wedges and serve hot.

Nutritional Facts (per serving)
CALORIES: 139 CARBOHYDRATES: 7 g CHOLESTEROL: 5 mg FAT: 5.4 g SAT. FAT: 1.7 g FIBER: 1.4 g PROTEIN: 16 g SODIUM: 514 mg CALCIUM: 142 mg
   Diabetic exchanges: 2 very lean meat, 1 vegetable, 1 fat

■ ■ ■

Ham & Pepper Frittata

YIELD: 4 SERVINGS

1 tablespoon extra virgin olive oil or canola oil

½ cup diced yellow bell pepper

½ cup diced green bell pepper

½ cup diced red bell pepper

1 cup diced, lean, reduced-sodium ham

2 teaspoons dried parsley

¼ teaspoon coarsely ground black pepper

2 cups fat-free egg substitute

1 cup shredded, reduced-fat, white cheddar or
   Swiss cheese

1. Coat a large ovenproof skillet with the olive oil and preheat over medium-high heat. Add the peppers, ham, parsley, and black pepper and sauté for several minutes, until the vegetables are crisp-tender and the ham is beginning to brown. Spread the mixture evenly over the bottom of the skillet.

2. Pour the egg substitute over the skillet mixture and reduce the heat to medium-low. Cover and cook without stirring for about 6 minutes, until the eggs are almost set (the edges will be cooked but the top will still be runny).

3. Remove the lid from the skillet and wrap the handle in aluminum foil (to prevent it from becoming damaged under the broiler). Place the skillet under a preheated broiler and broil for a couple of minutes, until the eggs are set but not dry. Sprinkle the cheese over the top and broil for another minute to melt the cheese. Cut the frittata into 4 wedges and serve hot.

Nutritional Facts (per serving)
CALORIES: 222 CARBOHYDRATES: 7 g
CHOLESTEROL: 32 mg FAT: 8.3 g SAT. FAT: 2.9 g
FIBER: 1.1 g PROTEIN: 28 g SODIUM: 690 mg
CALCIUM: 299 mg
   Diabetic exchanges: 4 lean meat, 1 vegetable, ½ fat

■ ■ ■

Southwestern Egg Scramble

YIELD: 4 SERVINGS

¾ cup canned (drained) hominy

2 tablespoons chopped green chilies

2 cups fat-free egg substitute

½ cup shredded, reduced-fat Monterey Jack (plain or with hot peppers) or Mexican cheese blend

1. Coat a large nonstick skillet with cooking spray and preheat over medium heat. Add the hominy to the skillet and cook for about 1 minute, until heated through.

2. Stir the chilies into the egg substitute and pour over the hominy. Reduce the heat to medium-low and cook without stirring for several minutes, until the eggs are set around the edges. Stirring gently to scramble, continue to cook for another minute, until the eggs are almost set.

3. Sprinkle the cheese over the eggs and cook just until the eggs are set but not dry and the cheese is melted. Serve hot.

Nutritional Facts (per serving)

CALORIES: 125 CARBOHYDRATES: 7 g CHOLESTEROL: 1 mg FAT: 2.3 g SAT. FAT: 1 g FIBER: 1 g PROTEIN: 17 g SODIUM: 414 mg CALCIUM: 169 mg

Diabetic exchanges: 2½ very lean meat, ½ starch

■ ■ ■

Potato & Egg Skillet

YIELD: 4 SERVINGS

5 cups shredded frozen (unthawed) hash brown potatoes

¼ cup chopped onion

¼ cup chopped green bell pepper

¼ teaspoon salt

Butter-flavored cooking spray

4 large eggs

¾ cup shredded reduced-fat cheddar cheese

1. Place the potatoes, onion, bell pepper, and salt in a large bowl and toss to mix well. Coat a large nonstick skillet with the cooking spray and spread the potato mixture loosely over the bottom of the skillet.

2. Place the skillet over medium heat, cover, and cook for 4 minutes, just until the potatoes are beginning to turn color on the bottom. Spray the tops of the potatoes with the cooking spray, turn them with a spatula (do not press or pack them down), and cook for 4 minutes more, until the potatoes are golden brown on the bottom.

3. Spray and turn the potatoes again, then reduce the heat under the skillet to medium-low. Make 4 wells in the potato mixture, spacing them evenly apart, and spray the bottom of the skillet in each well with cooking spray. Break an egg into each well. Cover the skillet

and cook for about 3 minutes, until the whites are firm and the yolks are beginning to thicken.

4. Sprinkle the cheese over the top, cover, and cook for an additional minute, or just until the cheese is melted. Serve hot.

Nutritional Facts (per serving)
CALORIES: 224 CARBOHYDRATES: 21 g
CHOLESTEROL: 201 mg FAT: 7 g SAT. FAT: 2.5 g
FIBER: 2.9 g PROTEIN: 16 g SODIUM: 408 mg
CALCIUM: 213 mg
   Diabetic exchanges: 2 medium-fat meat, 1¼ starch

■ ■ ■

Southwestern Egg Sandwich

YIELD: 1 SERVING

1 tablespoon canned chopped green chilies

¼ cup fat-free egg substitute

1 slice turkey bacon, cooked

1 slice (¾ ounce) reduced-fat Monterey Jack or cheddar cheese

1 whole-wheat or oat-bran English muffin, toasted

1 tablespoon salsa (optional)

1. Coat a medium-sized nonstick skillet with cooking spray and preheat over medium heat.

2. Stir the chilies into the egg substitute, then pour the mixture into the skillet. Cook without stirring for a minute or two, until the eggs are set around the edges. Use a spatula to lift the edges of the eggs and allow the un-

cooked egg to flow underneath the cooked portion. Cook for another minute, until the eggs are almost set. Fold the eggs in half, then fold in half again (so it will fit on the English muffin).

3. Break the bacon slice in half, lay it over the eggs, and then top with the cheese slice. Reduce the heat to low, cover and cook for another 30 seconds, until the cheese begins to melt. Place the egg, bacon, and cheese on the bottom half of the English muffin. Top with the salsa if desired, cover with the top half of the muffin, and serve hot.

Nutritional Facts (per serving)
CALORIES: 249 CARBOHYDRATES: 28 g
CHOLESTEROL: 21 mg FAT: 5.2 g SAT. FAT: 2 g
FIBER: 4.6 g PROTEIN: 22 g SODIUM: 842 mg
CALCIUM: 384 mg
   Diabetic exchanges: 2½ lean meat, 2 starch

■ ■ ■

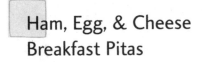

Ham, Egg, & Cheese Breakfast Pitas

YIELD: 4 SERVINGS

¾ cup sliced fresh mushrooms

¼ cup sliced scallions

½ cup diced lean ham

1 cup fat-free egg substitute

½ cup shredded, reduced-fat cheddar cheese

2 pieces whole-wheat or oat-bran pita bread (6-inch rounds), cut in half

1. Coat a large nonstick skillet with cooking spray and place over medium-high heat. Add the mushrooms, scallions, and ham and sauté for a couple of minutes, until the vegetables are tender and the ham is lightly browned.

2. Reduce the heat to medium-low and pour the egg substitute over the skillet mixture. Cook without stirring for a minute or two, until the eggs are set around the edges. Using a wooden spoon or spatula, begin pushing the eggs to the center of the skillet and stir gently to scramble. Cook just until the eggs are set but not dry. Remove the skillet from the heat, sprinkle the cheese over the top, and let it sit for a minute to melt the cheese.

3. Place the pitas on a large plate, cover with a paper towel, and microwave for about 20 seconds to heat through. Fill each pita half with a quarter of the egg mixture and serve hot.

Nutritional Facts (per serving)

CALORIES: 159 CARBOHYDRATES: 18 g
CHOLESTEROL: 21 mg FAT: 2.8 g SAT. FAT: 1.1 g
FIBER: 4.6 g PROTEIN: 17 g SODIUM: 535 mg
CALCIUM: 172 mg

Diabetic exchanges: 2 lean meat, 1 starch

■ ■ ■

Eggs Benedict Con Queso

For variety, substitute 1¼ cup of cooked crabmeat or shrimp for the Canadian bacon or ham.

YIELD: 5 SERVINGS

5 large eggs
5 slices (1 ounce each) Canadian bacon or
   lean ham
5 whole-wheat or oat-bran English muffin
   halves, toasted
3 tablespoons chopped fresh cilantro or thinly
   sliced scallions

SAUCE

1 tablespoon unbleached flour
¾ cup nonfat or low-fat milk
¾ cup diced reduced-fat process cheese (like
   Velveeta Light)
¼ cup chunky-style salsa

1. To poach the eggs, fill a large nonstick skillet with 3 inches of water and bring the water to a boil over high heat. Reduce the heat to low to keep the water gently simmering. Break the eggs, one at a time, into a custard cup. Holding the cup at the water's surface, slip the eggs, one at a time, into the water, spacing them evenly apart. Cover the skillet and cook for several minutes, or until the whites are completely set and the yolks

thicken. Lift the eggs out of the water with a slotted spoon, set aside, and keep warm.

2. To make the sauce, combine the flour and a couple tablespoons of the milk in a 1½-quart microwave-safe bowl and whisk until smooth. Whisk in the remaining milk. Microwave at high power for 1 minute, stir, and cook for another minute or until thick and bubbly. Stir in the cheese and cook in the microwave for another minute to melt the cheese and then stir in the salsa and heat for about 30 seconds. Set aside.

3. Coat a large nonstick skillet with nonstick cooking spray and preheat over medium-high heat. Add the Canadian bacon or ham to the skillet and cook for about 1 minute on each side, or until lightly browned.

4. To assemble the dish, place one English muffin half on each of 5 serving plates. Top each muffin half with 1 slice of Canadian bacon and 1 egg. Spoon one-fifth of the sauce over each serving and sprinkle with some of the cilantro or scallions. Serve hot.

Nutritional Facts (per serving)

CALORIES: 225 CARBOHYDRATES: 19 g
CHOLESTEROL: 224 mg FAT: 7.5 g SAT. FAT: 2.3 g
FIBER: 2.5 g PROTEIN: 20 g SODIUM: 804 mg
CALCIUM: 302 mg

   Diabetic exchanges: 2½ lean meat, 1 starch

■ ■ ■

Berry Breakfast Parfait

YIELD: 1 SERVING

8 ounces light vanilla yogurt
½ cup fresh raspberries, blueberries, sliced strawberries, or mixed fresh berries
¼ cup low-fat granola

1. Place 1½ tablespoons of the yogurt in the bottom of a 10-ounce balloon wine glass or parfait glass. Top the yogurt with half of the berries, half of the remaining yogurt, and half of the granola.

2. Repeat the layers and serve immediately.

Nutritional Facts (per serving)

CALORIES: 241 CARBOHYDRATES: 45 g
CHOLESTEROL: 5 mg FAT: 1.4 g SAT. FAT: 0.3 g FIBER: 4 g
PROTEIN: 12 g SODIUM: 215 mg CALCIUM: 379 mg

   Diabetic exchanges: 1 fruit, 1 starch, 1⅓ low-fat milk

■ ■ ■

Breakfast Banana Split

YIELD: 1 SERVING

½ small banana
6 ounces light vanilla yogurt
½ cup sliced strawberries or mixed fresh berries
2 tablespoons sliced almonds, low-fat granola, or honey crunch wheat germ

1. Cut the banana in half lengthwise and lay in the bottom of a medium-sized bowl.

2. Top the banana with the yogurt, berries, almonds, and granola or wheat germ. Serve immediately.

Nutritional Facts (per serving)

CALORIES: 245 CARBOHYDRATES: 36 g
CHOLESTEROL: 4 mg FAT: 7 g SAT. FAT: 0.6 g FIBER: 4.5 g
PROTEIN: 11 g SODIUM: 125 mg CALCIUM: 305 mg
   Diabetic exchanges: 1½ fruit, 1 low-fat milk, 1 fat

■ ■ ■

Frosty Fruit Smoothie

YIELD: 1 SERVING

1 cup nonfat or low-fat milk
1 packet sugar-free vanilla Carnation Instant Breakfast
¾ cup unsweetened frozen blueberries or sliced peaches
½ cup unsweetened frozen raspberries

1. Put all of the ingredients in a blender and blend until smooth.

2. Pour into a tall glass and serve immediately.

Nutritional Facts (per 2-cup serving)

CALORIES: 236 CARBOHYDRATES: 42 g
CHOLESTEROL: 7 mg FAT: 1 g SAT. FAT: 0.4 g FIBER: 5.9 g
PROTEIN: 15 g SODIUM: 234 mg CALCIUM: 719 mg
   Diabetic exchanges: 2 low-fat milk, 1¼ fruit

■ ■ ■

Rolled Swedish Pancakes

For variety, substitute coarsely chopped light apple pie filling for the cherry pie filling.

YIELD: 6 SERVINGS

¾ cup oat-bran
½ cup whole-wheat pastry flour
1½ tablespoons sugar substitute or sugar
1 tablespoon baking powder
¾ teaspoon dried grated lemon rind
1¾ cups nonfat or low-fat milk
1¼ cups fat-free egg substitute
1½ cups sugar-free or light (reduced-sugar) cherry pie filling
¾ cup nonfat or light sour cream
⅓ cup chopped walnuts

1. Preheat oven to 200°.

2. Place the oat-bran, flour, ½ tablespoon of the sugar substitute or sugar, baking powder, and lemon rind in a medium-sized bowl and stir to mix well. Add the milk and egg substitute and stir with a wire whisk until smooth. (The batter will be thin.)

3. Coat a large griddle or nonstick skillet with nonstick cooking spray and preheat over medium heat until a drop of water sizzles when it hits the heated surface. (If using an electric griddle, heat the griddle according to the manufacturer's directions.)

4. For each pancake, pour ¼ cup of the

batter onto the griddle or skillet (the mixture will spread out to form a 6-inch circle). Cook for about 1½ minutes, until the top is bubbly and the edges are dry. Turn and cook for an additional minute, until the second side is golden brown. Repeat until all of the batter is used up, respraying the griddle or skillet as necessary.

5. As the pancakes are done, roll them up, place them on a serving plate, and keep warm in a preheated oven.

6. To assemble the pancakes, place the sour cream and remaining sugar substitute or sugar in a small bowl and stir to mix well. Set aside. Unroll a pancake and spread 2 table-spoons of the pie filling along one end. Reroll the pancake to enclose the filling and place on a serving plate. Repeat with the remaining in-gredients to make 12 filled pancakes. Serve hot, topping each serving with some of the sour cream mixture and a sprinkling of walnuts.

Nutritional Facts (per 2-pancake serving)
CALORIES: 238 CARBOHYDRATES: 34 g
CHOLESTEROL: 6 mg FAT: 6.6 g SAT. FAT: 1.7 g
FIBER: 4.2 g PROTEIN: 13.4 g SODIUM: 418 mg
CALCIUM: 252 mg
   Diabetic exchanges: 1 very lean meat, 1 starch, 1 fruit, ¼ low-fat milk, 1 fat

■ ■ ■

Creamy Cheese Grits

The addition of milk and cheese to this Southern breakfast favorite packs in protein and extra calcium.

YIELD: 5 SERVINGS

¾ cup quick-cooking corn grits (look for the
   kind that cooks in 5 minutes)
1½ cups nonfat or low-fat milk
1½ cups water
1 cup finely diced or shredded reduced-fat
   process cheese (like Velveeta Light)

1. Place the grits, milk, and water in a 2-quart pot and bring to a boil over medium-high heat. Reduce the heat to low, cover, and simmer, stirring frequently, for about 5 min-utes, until the grits are tender.

2. Add the cheese and cook uncovered, stirring constantly for about 3 minutes more, until the cheese is melted and the mixture is thick. Serve hot.

Nutritional Facts (per ¾-cup serving)
CALORIES: 154 CARBOHYDRATES: 23 g CHOLESTEROL: 11 mg FAT: 2.8 g SAT. FAT: 1.7 g FIBER: 1.2 g PROTEIN: 9 g SODIUM: 397 mg CALCIUM: 220 mg
   Diabetic exchanges: 1 lean meat, 1 starch, ⅓ low-fat milk

■ ■ ■

Double Bran Muffins

YIELD: 12 MUFFINS

1 cup oat-bran

1 cup wheat bran

¼ cup brown sugar

2 teaspoons baking powder

1 cup nonfat or low-fat milk

¼ cup fat-free egg substitute or 2 egg
   whites, beaten

¼ cup molasses or honey

2 tablespoons canola oil

½ cup chopped walnuts, pecans, raisins, or
   chopped dried fruit (or any combination)
   (optional)

1. Preheat oven to 350°.

2. Place the oat bran, wheat bran, and brown sugar in a medium bowl and stir to mix well. Use the back of a spoon to press out the lumps in the brown sugar. Add the baking powder and stir to mix well.

3. Combine the milk, egg substitute or egg whites, molasses or honey, and oil and stir to mix. Add the milk mixture to the bran mixture and stir to mix well. Fold in the nuts and/or dried fruits if desired.

4. Coat the bottoms only of muffin cups with nonstick cooking spray and divide the batter among the muffin cups. Bake at 350 degrees for about 15 minutes, until a wooden

toothpick inserted in the center of a muffin comes out clean.

5. Remove the muffin tin from the oven and allow it to sit for 5 minutes before removing the muffins. Serve warm or at room temperature.

Nutritional Facts (per 1 muffin)
CALORIES: 94 CARBOHYDRATES: 18 g
CHOLESTEROL: 0 mg FAT: 3 g SAT. FAT: 0.3 g FIBER: 3.3 g
PROTEIN: 3.3 g SODIUM: 105 mg CALCIUM: 95 mg
   Diabetic exchanges: 1 starch, ¼ other carbohydrate, ½ fat

■ ■ ■

Hot & Hearty Oat Bran

This nutritious, high-fiber alternative to cream of wheat cooks in just 2 minutes.

YIELD: 1 SERVING

½ cup oat bran

¾ cup nonfat or low-fat milk

½ cup water

1½ tablespoons raisins or chopped dried fruit

1 tablespoon sliced almonds

1. Place the oat bran, milk, and water in a microwave safe bowl and stir to mix well. Microwave at high power for about 2 to 3 minutes, until thick and creamy.

2. Serve hot topped with the raisins and

almonds. Top with additional milk and a drizzle of honey or maple syrup or some artificial sweetener if desired. Serve immediately.

Nutritional Facts (per serving)
CALORIES: 254 CARBOHYDRATES: 51 g
CHOLESTEROL: 0 mg FAT: 6.7 g SAT. FAT: 1.1 g
FIBER: 8.7 g PROTEIN: 16 g SODIUM: 101 mg
CALCIUM: 272 mg
   Diabetic exchanges: 2 starch, ¾ fruit, ¾ low-fat milk, 1 fat

■ ■ ■

Toasted Muesli

YIELD: 8 SERVINGS

2 cups old-fashioned oats (the kind that cook in 5 minutes)
¾ cup sliced almonds or chopped pecans
¾ cup chopped dried apricots, raisins, or mixed dried fruit
1 cup All Bran or Fiber One cereal
½ cup honey crunch wheat germ

1. Preheat oven to 350°.

2. Spread the oats and nuts over a large baking sheet. Bake for about 7 minutes, stirring once, until the nuts are lightly toasted (be careful not to let them burn). Let them cool to room temperature.

3. Place the oat mixture in a large bowl. Add the dried fruit, bran cereal, and wheat germ and stir to mix well. Transfer to an airtight container and store for up to 1 month.

4. To serve, place ½ cup of the muesli in a serving bowl. Add ¾ cup nonfat or low-fat milk or light vanilla yogurt. Stir and let sit for 5 minutes before serving.

Nutritional Facts (per serving, cereal only)
CALORIES: 201 CARBOHYDRATES: 32 g
CHOLESTEROL: 0 mg FAT: 7 g SAT. FAT: 0.7 g FIBER: 8.3 g
PROTEIN: 8.3 g SODIUM: 33 mg CALCIUM: 66 mg
   Diabetic exchanges: 1½ starch, ½ fruit, 1 fat

■ ■ ■

9. PARTY PLEASING HORS D'OEUVRES

There's no doubt about it. Great food helps make any get-together better. Unfortunately, this often means going all out—and piling on extra fat, calories, and carbs. However, with just a little imagination, you can easily whip up an assortment of creative and delicious snacks and never stray from your light and healthy lifestyle.

Can party foods be healthy *and* special enough to serve to guests? Absolutely. Ingredients like low-fat cheese, ultra-lean meats, low-fat sour cream, and light mayonnaise can dramatically trim fat and calories from traditional party favorites. "Good carbs" like wholesome whole-grain crackers, hearty breads, and whole-wheat tortilla wraps can also star in a variety of festive recipes. This chapter combines these ingredients plus plenty of fresh vegetables and fruits to create a variety of delectable hot and cold hors d'oeuvres that are sure to perk up any party.

Smoked Salmon Canapés

YIELD: 24 APPETIZERS

6 slices firm pumpernickel or whole-wheat bread
¼ cup plus 2 tablespoons light vegetable-
  flavored cream cheese spread
4 ounces thinly sliced smoked salmon, cut into
  1½-inch pieces
½ cup peeled, seeded, and finely chopped
  cucumber
24 small sprigs fresh dill or 1 teaspoon dried dill

1. Trim the crusts from the bread slices and spread each slice with 1 tablespoon of the cream cheese.

2. Cut each bread slice diagonally into quarters to make 4 triangles. Top each triangle with a folded piece of salmon, a teaspoon of cucumber, and a sprig of fresh dill or a small pinch of dried dill. Serve immediately. (To make in advance, top the canapés with the cream cheese and salmon. Cover with plastic wrap and chill for up to 3 hours before serving. Add the cucumber and dill just before serving.)

Nutritional Facts (per appetizer)
CALORIES: 31 CARBOHYDRATES: 4 g CHOLESTEROL: 5 mg
FAT: 0.9 g SAT. FAT: 0.3 g FIBER: 0.5 g PROTEIN: 2 g
SODIUM: 140 mg CALCIUM: 8 mg
   Diabetic exchanges: ¼ starch, ⅓ lean meat

■ ■ ■

Marinated Artichoke Appetizers

YIELD: 24 APPETIZERS

24 marinated artichoke quarters, drained
24 cherry or grape tomatoes
8-ounce block reduced-fat white cheddar or
  Swiss cheese, cut into 24 cubes

1. Skewer one artichoke piece, tomato, and cheese cube onto a toothpick.

2. Serve immediately or cover and refrigerate until ready to serve.

Nutritional Facts (per appetizer)
CALORIES: 37 CARBOHYDRATES: 1.8 g
CHOLESTEROL: 5 mg FAT: 2.1 g SAT. FAT: 0.6 g
FIBER: 0.7 g PROTEIN: 3 g SODIUM: 92 mg
CALCIUM: 84 mg
   Diabetic exchanges: ⅓ medium-fat meat, ⅓ vegetable

■ ■ ■

Turkey & Vegetable Wrappetizers

YIELD: 28 APPETIZERS

Olive oil cooking spray
12 thin asparagus spears
Pinch dried thyme

4 whole-wheat or spinach flour tortillas (10-inch
rounds)

1 cup light vegetable-flavored cream cheese
spread

8 ounces thinly sliced roasted turkey breast

8 strips roasted red bell pepper (each about
1 by 4 inches)

1. Preheat oven to 450°.

2. Coat a medium baking sheet with cooking spray and spread the asparagus spears in an even layer over the bottom of the pan. Spray the top of the asparagus lightly with the cooking spray and sprinkle with the thyme. Bake uncovered for 8 to 10 minutes, until tender and lightly browned. Set aside to cool to room temperature (or make the day before and refrigerate until ready to assemble the appetizers).

3. Spread each tortilla with ¼ cup of the cream cheese, extending it all the way to the outer edges. Lay a quarter of the turkey over the bottom half only of each tortilla, leaving a 1-inch margin on each outer edge. Lay 3 asparagus spears and 2 bell pepper strips along the lower edge of the tortilla.

4. Starting at the bottom, roll each tortilla up tightly. Cut a 1¼-inch piece off each end, and discard. Slice the remainder of each tortilla into seven 1-inch pieces. Arrange the rolls on a platter and serve immediately. Or wrap the rolls in plastic wrap and refrigerate for several hours before slicing and serving.

Nutritional Facts (per appetizer)
CALORIES: 42 CARBOHYDRATES: 5 g CHOLESTEROL: 8 mg
FAT: 1.5 g SAT. FAT: 0.6 g FIBER: 0.5 g PROTEIN: 2.7 g
SODIUM: 118 mg CALCIUM: 6 mg
  Diabetic exchanges: ¼ starch, ¼ lean meat

■ ■ ■

Sun-Dried Tomato & Artichoke Pizzas

YIELD: 24 APPETIZERS

4 whole-wheat or oat-bran pita pockets (6-inch
rounds)

¼ cup chopped sun-dried tomatoes packed in
olive oil, drained

1 cup chopped canned or marinated artichoke
hearts, well drained

1 cup shredded reduced-fat mozzarella cheese

1. Preheat oven to 400°.

2. Arrange the pitas on a large baking sheet and scatter a quarter of the sun-dried tomatoes and artichoke hearts over each one, and top with some of the cheese.

3. Bake for about 8 minutes, until the cheese is melted and lightly browned. Cut each pizza into 6 wedges and serve hot.

Nutritional Facts (per appetizer)

CALORIES: 40 CARBOHYDRATES: 6 g CHOLESTEROL: 2 mg
FAT: 1.1 g SAT. FAT: 0.5 g FIBER: 1.1 g PROTEIN: 2.5 g
SODIUM: 82 mg CALCIUM: 44 mg

Diabetic exchanges: ⅓ starch, ⅙ medium-fat meat

■ ■ ■

Pesto Party Pizzas

YIELD: 24 APPETIZERS

4 whole-wheat or oat-bran pita pockets (6-inch
rounds)
3 to 4 tablespoons prepared pesto
2 medium-small plum tomatoes, thinly sliced
1 cup shredded reduced-fat mozzarella cheese

1. Preheat oven to 400°.

2. Arrange the pitas on a large baking
sheet and spread each one with a quarter of
the pesto. Top with a quarter of the tomato
slices, and a quarter of the cheese. Bake for
about 8 minutes, until the cheese is melted
and lightly browned. Cut each pizza into 6
wedges and serve hot.

Nutritional Facts (per appetizer)

CALORIES: 45 CARBOHYDRATES: 5 g CHOLESTEROL: 3 mg
FAT: 1.8 g SAT. FAT: 0.7 g FIBER: 0.8 g PROTEIN: 2.7 g
SODIUM: 90 mg CALCIUM: 55 mg

Diabetic exchanges: ⅓ starch, ⅙ medium-fat meat

■ ■ ■

Spinach and Sun-Dried Tomato Quesadillas

YIELD: 16 APPETIZERS

2 tablespoons julienned or diced sun-dried
tomatoes in olive oil, drained
1½ cups (moderately packed) chopped fresh
spinach
1 cup shredded nonfat or reduced-fat
mozzarella cheese
4 whole-wheat flour tortillas (8-inch rounds)

1. Place 1 to 2 teaspoons of the oil from
the jar of sun-dried tomatoes in a medium
nonstick skillet and place over medium-high
heat. Add the spinach and sauté for a minute
or two, just until the spinach is wilted. Remove the skillet from the heat and stir in the
sun-dried tomatoes.

2. Lay a tortilla on a flat surface and
sprinkle the *bottom half only* with a quarter of
the spinach mixture. Sprinkle with a quarter
of the cheese. Fold the top half of the tortilla
over to enclose the filling. Repeat with the remaining ingredients to make 4 filled tortillas.

3. Coat a large griddle or nonstick skillet
with nonstick cooking spray and preheat over
medium heat until a drop of water sizzles
when it hits the heated surface.

4. Lay the quesadillas on the griddle and
cook for about 1½ minutes, until the bottoms are golden brown. Spray the tops lightly

with the cooking spray and then turn with a spatula. Cook for an additional 1½ minutes, until the second side is golden brown.

5. Transfer the quesadillas to a cutting board and cut each one into 4 wedges. Serve hot.

_____

Nutritional Facts (per appetizer)

CALORIES: 47 CARBOHYDRATES: 7 g CHOLESTEROL: 1 mg FAT: 0.9 g SAT. FAT: 0 g FIBER: 0.9 g PROTEIN: 3 g SODIUM: 142 mg CALCIUM: 106 mg

Diabetic exchanges: ½ starch, ¼ medium-fat meat

■ ■ ■

Black Bean Quesadillas

YIELD: 16 APPETIZERS

1 cup canned, drained black beans

1 teaspoon chili powder

2 tablespoons canned chopped green chilies

4 whole-wheat flour tortillas (8-inch rounds)

1 cup shredded nonfat or reduced-fat Mexican blend or Monterey Jack cheese

¼ cup nonfat or light sour cream

2 tablespoons chopped fresh tomatoes or chunky-style salsa

2 tablespoons chopped fresh cilantro or sliced scallions

1. Combine the beans and chili powder in a small bowl and mash with a fork. Stir in the green chilies.

2. Lay a tortilla on a flat surface and sprin-kle the *bottom half only* with 2 tablespoons of the cheese. Top the cheese with a quarter of the bean mixture and 2 more tablespoons of cheese. Fold the top half of the tortilla over to enclose the filling. Repeat with the remaining ingredients to make 4 filled tortillas.

3. Coat a large griddle or nonstick skillet with nonstick cooking spray and preheat over medium heat until a drop of water sizzles when it hits the heated surface.

4. Lay the quesadillas on the griddle and cook for about 1½ minutes, or until the bottoms are golden brown. Spray the tops lightly with the cooking spray and then turn with a spatula. Cook for an additional 1½ minutes, or until the second side is golden brown.

5. Transfer the quesadillas to a cutting board and cut each one into 4 wedges. Serve hot accompanied by the sour cream, tomatoes or salsa, and cilantro or scallions.

_____

Nutritional Facts (per appetizer)

CALORIES: 57 CARBOHYDRATES: 9 g CHOLESTEROL: 1 mg FAT: 1 g SAT. FAT: 0.1 g FIBER: 1.4 g PROTEIN: 4 g SODIUM: 195 mg CALCIUM: 73 mg

Diabetic exchanges: ½ starch, ½ very lean meat

■ ■ ■

Simple Veggie Skewers

YIELD: 12 APPETIZERS

1 medium-small zucchini squash
12 cubes (¾-inches each) reduced-fat white
   cheddar, provolone, or Swiss cheese (about
   3 ounces)
12 small whole fresh mushrooms
12 pitted jumbo black olives
12 cherry or grape tomatoes
12 wooden skewers (6-inches each)
½ cup light ranch salad dressing (optional)

1. Trim the ends off the zucchini, quarter it lengthwise, and cut into ¾-inch pieces.

2. Thread 1 of the zucchini pieces, 1 cube of cheese, 1 mushroom, 1 olive, 1 tomato, and another zucchini piece onto each skewer. Serve immediately (accompanied by the dressing if desired) or cover and chill for several hours before serving.

Nutritional Facts (per appetizer)
CALORIES: 58 CARBOHYDRATES: 2 g CHOLESTEROL: 7 mg FAT: 2.8 g SAT. FAT: 1 g FIBER: 1 g PROTEIN: 5 g SODIUM: 138 mg CALCIUM: 130 mg
   Diabetic exchanges: ½ vegetable, ½ medium-fat meat

■ ■ ■

Stuffed Celery with Apples & Cheese

YIELD: 48 APPETIZERS

8-ounce block light (Neufchâtel) cream cheese
1 large Granny Smith apple, peeled and very
   finely chopped (about 1 cup)
½ cup shredded reduced-fat cheddar cheese
¼ cup finely chopped dates
¼ cup finely chopped walnuts
48 pieces celery (2 inches each)

1. To make the filling, place the cream cheese, apples, cheese, dates, and walnuts in a medium bowl and beat to mix well. Cover and chill for at least 1 hour.

2. Pipe or spoon about 2 teaspoons of the filling into each piece of celery. Serve immediately.

Nutritional Facts (per 3 appetizers)
CALORIES: 74 CARBOHYDRATES: 5 g CHOLESTEROL: 12 mg FAT: 4.7 g SAT. FAT: 2.4 g FIBER: 1 g PROTEIN: 3.4 g SODIUM: 109 mg CALCIUM: 56 mg
   Diabetic exchanges: ⅓ fruit, 1 fat

■ ■ ■

Turkey & Cream Cheese Roll-ups

YIELD: 16 APPETIZERS

16 thin round slices (about 3½ inches) roasted
    turkey breast (about 7 ounces)
½ cup scallion & chives or vegetable-flavored
    light cream cheese
32 fresh baby spinach or arugula leaves

1. Lay a slice of turkey out on a flat surface and spread ½ tablespoon of the cream cheese and 2 spinach or arugula leaves over *the bottom only* of the slice. Roll the slice up to enclose the filling and secure with a wooden toothpick. Repeat with the remaining ingredients to make 16 roll-ups.

2. Arrange the roll-ups on a lettuce-lined platter and serve immediately, or cover and chill until ready to serve.

Nutritional Facts (per appetizer)
CALORIES: 27 CARBOHYDRATES: 1 g CHOLESTEROL: 10 mg
FAT: 1.4 g SAT. FAT: 0.7 g FIBER: 0 g PROTEIN: 3 g
SODIUM: 138 mg CALCIUM: 8 mg
   Diabetic exchanges: ½ lean meat

■ ■ ■

Crab Louis Dip

YIELD: 2 CUPS

½ cup nonfat or light mayonnaise
½ cup light sour cream
3 tablespoons chili sauce
¾ cup cooked flaked crabmeat or 1 can
    (6 ounces) crabmeat, drained
¼ cup chopped black or green olives
1½ tablespoons finely chopped scallions

1. Combine the mayonnaise, sour cream, and chili sauce in a medium bowl and stir to mix. Stir in the remaining ingredients.

2. Cover and chill for at least 2 hours. Serve with whole-grain crackers, celery sticks, and carrot sticks.

Nutritional Facts (per 2-tablespoon serving)
CALORIES: 26 CARBOHYDRATES: 2 g CHOLESTEROL: 8 mg
FAT: 1 g SAT. FAT: 0.6 g FIBER: 0.1 g PROTEIN: 2 g
SODIUM: 134 mg CALCIUM: 18 mg
   Diabetic exchanges: ¼ lean meat

■ ■ ■

Smoked Salmon Spread

YIELD: ABOUT 2 CUPS

8-ounce block light (Neufchâtel) cream cheese
¼ cup nonfat or light mayonnaise
1 cup flaked smoked salmon
2 tablespoons finely chopped scallions
½ to 1 tablespoon finely chopped fresh dill or
    ½ to 1 teaspoon dried dill (optional)

1. Place the cream cheese in a medium bowl and beat for about 1 minute. Add the mayonnaise and beat to mix well. Stir in the remaining ingredients.

2. Serve with whole-grain crackers and fresh-cut vegetables or use to fill hollowed-out cherry tomatoes or celery sticks.

Nutritional Facts (per 2-tablespoon serving)
CALORIES: 48 CARBOHYDRATES: 1 g CHOLESTEROL: 12 mg
FAT: 3.4 g SAT. FAT: 2 g FIBER: 0 g PROTEIN: 3 g
SODIUM: 152 mg CALCIUM: 12 mg
Diabetic exchanges: ½ medium-fat meat

■ ■ ■

Scallion & Olive Hummus

YIELD: ABOUT 1¾ CUPS

16-ounce can garbanzo beans
¼ cup sesame tahini
1 tablespoon plus 1 teaspoon lemon juice
2 teaspoons extra virgin olive oil
2 teaspoons crushed garlic
½ teaspoon ground cumin
¼ teaspoon coarsely ground black pepper
¼ cup (packed) chopped fresh parsley
⅓ to ½ cup sliced scallions
½ cup coarsely chopped black olives

1. Drain the beans, reserving 2 tablespoons of the liquid. Place the beans, tahini, lemon juice, olive oil, garlic, cumin, pepper, and 1 tablespoon of the reserved liquid in the bowl of a food processor and process until smooth.

2. Add the parsley and scallions and process until finely chopped. Add the olives and process until the olives are finely chopped. Add a little more of the reserved liquid if the mixture seems too thick.

3. Serve immediately with wedges of warm whole-grain pita bread or whole-grain crackers and celery sticks, or cover and refrigerate until ready to serve.

Nutritional Facts (per 2-tablespoon serving)
CALORIES: 62 CARBOHYDRATES: 6 g CHOLESTEROL: 0 mg
FAT: 3.8 g SAT. FAT: 0.4 g FIBER: 1.6 g PROTEIN: 2.2 g
SODIUM: 126 mg CALCIUM: 22 mg
Diabetic exchanges: ⅓ starch, ⅓ lean meat

■ ■ ■

FIBER: 0.4 g PROTEIN: 6.5 g SODIUM: 143 mg
CALCIUM: 70 mg
Diabetic exchanges: 1 medium-fat meat

▪ ▪ ▪

Pesto Cheese Log

YIELD: 8 SERVINGS

COATING

½ cup (moderately packed) fresh basil or cilantro

¼ cup (moderately packed) fresh parsley

¼ cup chopped walnuts or pine nuts

2 tablespoons grated Parmesan cheese

1½ teaspoons extra virgin olive oil

1 teaspoon crushed garlic

8 ounces soft-curd farmer cheese or soft goat cheese

1. Make sure the herbs are completely dry. Place all of the coating ingredients in a food processor and process, pulsing the food processor for several seconds at a time, until the mixture is finely ground. Set aside.

2. Shape the cheese into two 4-inch logs. Spread the pesto out on a sheet of waxed paper and roll the cheese logs in the pesto, gently pressing the pesto onto the logs to make it stick.

3. Serve immediately or cover and refrigerate until ready to serve. Serve with fresh cut vegetables, whole-grain crackers, wedges of whole-wheat or oat-bran pita bread, or small slices of sourdough bread.

Nutritional Facts (per serving)
CALORIES: 86 CARBOHYDRATES: 0.8 g
CHOLESTEROL: 11 mg FAT: 5.9 g SAT. FAT: 2 g

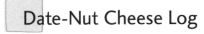

Date-Nut Cheese Log

For variety, substitute dried cranberries or cherries for the dates.

YIELD: 8 SERVINGS

COATING

½ cup chopped pitted dates

½ cup chopped walnuts

8 ounces soft-curd farmer cheese or soft goat cheese

1. Place the dates in the bowl of a food processor and process, pulsing the food processor for several seconds at a time, until the dates are very finely chopped. Add the walnuts and process for several seconds more, or until the walnuts are finely ground. Set aside.

2. Shape the cheese into two 4-inch logs. Spread the coating mixture out on a sheet of waxed paper and roll the cheese logs in the coating, gently pressing the coating onto the logs to make it stick.

3. Serve immediately or cover and refrigerate until ready to serve. Serve with fresh apple slices (dip the slices in pineapple juice to prevent browning), celery sticks, whole-grain crackers,

wedges of firm multigrain or pumpernickel bread, or thin slices of whole-grain bagels.

Nutritional Facts (per serving)
CALORIES: 125 CARBOHYDRATES: 9 g CHOLESTEROL: 9 mg FAT: 6.8 g SAT. FAT: 1.7 g FIBER: 1.2 g PROTEIN: 7 g SODIUM: 114 mg CALCIUM: 46 mg
Diabetic exchanges: ½ fruit, 1 medium-fat meat

■ ■ ■

Spicy Spinach & Artichoke Spread

YIELD: ABOUT 3 CUPS

10 ounces frozen chopped spinach, thawed and squeezed very dry
14-ounce can artichoke hearts, drained and finely chopped
8 ounces vegetable-flavored light cream cheese spread
½ cup nonfat or light mayonnaise
1 cup shredded Monterey Jack cheese with hot peppers (or use plain Monterey Jack for a milder flavor)
¼ cup grated Parmesan cheese

1. Preheat oven to 400°.
2. Place the spinach, artichoke hearts, cream cheese, mayonnaise, and half of the Monterey Jack and Parmesan cheeses in a medium bowl and stir to mix well.
3. Coat a 9-inch pie pan with nonstick cooking spray and spread the mixture evenly

in the pan. Cover with aluminum foil and bake for 20 minutes.

4. Remove the foil and top with the remaining Parmesan and Monterey Jack cheeses. Bake uncovered for an additional 5 minutes. Serve warm with low-fat tortilla chips or whole-grain crackers.

Nutritional Facts (per 2-tablespoon serving)
CALORIES: 50 CARBOHYDRATES: 2 g CHOLESTEROL: 10 mg FAT: 2.6 g SAT. FAT: 1.6 g FIBER: 1 g PROTEIN: 3.4 g SODIUM: 144 mg CALCIUM: 82 mg
Diabetic exchanges: ¼ vegetable, ¼ medium-fat meat

■ ■ ■

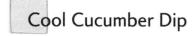

Cool Cucumber Dip

YIELD: 2 CUPS

1 medium-large cucumber, peeled, seeded, and chopped
¼ cup finely chopped sweet onion
1¼ cups light sour cream
3 tablespoons finely chopped fresh cilantro
½ teaspoon ground cumin
⅛ teaspoon salt
⅛ teaspoon ground white pepper

1. Place the cucumber in the bowl of a food processor and process until finely chopped. Roll the cucumber in several layers of cheesecloth or paper towels and squeeze out the excess moisture, discarding the liquid.

2. Place the chopped cucumber in a medium-sized bowl, add the remaining ingredients, and stir to mix well.

3. Serve immediately with low-fat tortilla chips and fresh-cut vegetables. Or transfer to a covered container and chill until ready to serve.

Nutritional Facts (per 2-tablespoon serving)
CALORIES: 27 CARBOHYDRATES: 2 g CHOLESTEROL: 6 mg FAT: 1.6 g SAT. FAT: 1.2 g FIBER: 0.1 g PROTEIN: 1.3 g SODIUM: 34 mg CALCIUM: 27 mg
Diabetic exchanges: ⅓ fat

■ ■ ■

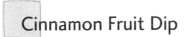

Cinnamon Fruit Dip

YIELD: 1⅛ CUPS

1 cup light sour cream
1½ tablespoons honey
1½ tablespoons sugar substitute
½ teaspoon ground cinnamon

1. Combine all of the ingredients in a small bowl and stir to mix well. Serve immediately or cover and chill until ready to serve.

2. Serve with fresh whole strawberries, pineapple chunks, apple and pear slices, and chunks of bananas. (Dip apple, pear, and banana pieces in pineapple juice to prevent browning.)

Nutritional Facts (per 2-tablespoon serving)
CALORIES: 46 CARBOHYDRATES: 4 g CHOLESTEROL: 8 mg FAT: 2.2 g SAT. FAT: 1.8 g FIBER: 0 g PROTEIN: 1.8 g SODIUM: 22 mg CALCIUM: 36 mg
Diabetic exchanges: ½ fat, ¼ other carbohydrate

■ ■ ■

Honey-Lime Fruit Dip

YIELD: ABOUT 1¼ CUPS

1 cup light sour cream
2 tablespoons honey
Sugar substitute equal to 2 tablespoons sugar
1½ tablespoons lime juice
1 teaspoon freshly grated lime rind

1. Combine all of the ingredients in a small bowl and stir to mix well. Serve immediately or cover and refrigerate until ready to serve.

2. Serve with fresh whole strawberries, cantaloupe and honeydew melon balls, and chunks of banana. (Dip banana pieces in pineapple juice to prevent browning.)

Nutritional Facts (per 2-tablespoon serving)
CALORIES: 46 CARBOHYDRATES: 5 g CHOLESTEROL: 8 mg FAT: 2 g SAT. FAT: 1.6 g FIBER: 0 g PROTEIN: 1.8 g SODIUM: 20 mg CALCIUM: 32 mg
Diabetic exchanges: ½ fat, ¼ other carbohydrate

■ ■ ■

Strawberries 'n Cream

YIELD: 24 APPETIZERS

12 large strawberries (about 12 ounces)
1 can pressurized whipped light cream
2 tablespoons shaved dark chocolate

1. Rinse the berries and pat dry with paper towels. Trim off the stem end and cut in half lengthwise. Cut a thin strip off the bottom of each berry half so they will sit upright without tipping over.

2. Squirt about 2 teaspoons of the whipped cream into the center of each berry and sprinkle about ¼ teaspoon of the chocolate over the top. Serve immediately, or cover and chill for up to 1 hour before serving.

Nutritional Facts (per 3 pieces)
CALORIES: 45 CARBOHYDRATES: 4.8 g CHOLESTEROL: 9 mg FAT: 3.3 g SAT. FAT: 1.8 g FIBER: 1.2 g PROTEIN: 0.6 g SODIUM: 3 mg CALCIUM: 12 mg
Diabetic exchanges: ⅓ fruit, ½ fat

■ ■ ■

10. HOT AND HEARTY SOUPS

Soups are perhaps the most versatile of foods, making them a real boon to the menu planner. A cup of soup is the perfect introduction to a meal or partner to a main dish salad or sandwich. A more substantial bowl of soup needs only a salad and piece of crusty whole-grain bread to make a satisfying lunch or light supper.

Made with light and healthy ingredients—such as lean meats, poultry, whole grains, beans, pasta, and plenty of garden vegetables—soup can be a boon to the weight watcher, too. Because soup contains a high proportion of water, you get a big serving for relatively few calories. This makes soup exceptionally filling and satisfying. Studies have even shown that people who eat soup for lunch tend to eat less later on in the day.

Even when you take the time to make soup from scratch, you'll find that soups are perfect for a busy lifestyle. Most soups can be prepared ahead of time and then refrigerated or frozen until needed. In fact, many soups taste even better when refrigerated overnight, allowing the flavors to blend.

This chapter combines wholesome ingredients to produce a variety of savory soups that are bursting with flavor and brimming with important nutrients. So take out your kettle and get ready to enjoy the warmth and comfort of a steaming bowl of soup.

Slow-cooked Beef, Barley, & Vegetable Soup

YIELD: 11 SERVINGS

1 ¼ pounds lean stew beef, cut into bite-
   size pieces
1 medium-large onion, cut into thin wedges
1 cup sliced carrot
1 tablespoon beef bouillon granules
1 ¼ teaspoons dried thyme
1 ¼ teaspoons dried oregano
¼ teaspoon ground black pepper
5 cups water
14 ½-ounce can diced tomatoes with
   roasted garlic
10 ¾-ounce can condensed tomato soup,
   undiluted
½ cup uncooked pearl barley
1 cup frozen green peas

1. Coat a large nonstick skillet with non-stick cooking spray and preheat over medium-high heat. Cook the beef in two batches for several minutes, until nicely browned.

2. Transfer the beef to a 3-quart or larger slow cooker. Add the onion, carrots, beef granules, thyme, oregano, and pepper. Pour in the water, undrained tomatoes, and tomato soup.

3. Cover and cook on high for 4 hours or on low for 8 hours. Add the barley and cook for an additional hour at high or 2 hours at low, until the barley is tender. Add the peas and cook for 30 minutes at high or 1 hour at low. Serve hot.

Nutritional Facts (per 1-cup serving)
CALORIES: 145 CARBOHYDRATES: 16 g
CHOLESTEROL: 29 mg FAT: 2.5 g SAT. FAT: 0.8 g
FIBER: 3 g PROTEIN: 14 g SODIUM: 442 mg
CALCIUM: 22 mg
   Diabetic exchanges: 1½ lean meat, ½ starch, 1½ vegetable

■ ■ ■

Italian Wedding Soup

YIELD: 6 SERVINGS

MEATBALLS
½ pound 95% lean ground beef or
   ground turkey
¼ cup very finely chopped onion
2 tablespoons fat-free egg substitute or 1 egg
   white, beaten
2 tablespoons oat bran
1 tablespoon grated Parmesan cheese
½ teaspoon dried Italian seasoning

5 cups unsalted chicken broth
¾ cup (¼-inch dice) carrots
2 teaspoons chicken bouillon granules
1 ½ teaspoons crushed garlic
2 cups thinly sliced escarole
½ cup uncooked orzo pasta or 3 ounces other
   small pasta

2 teaspoons dried parsley, finely crumbled

grated Parmesan cheese (optional)

1. To make the meatballs, combine all of the meatball ingredients and mix well. Shape into ¾-inch balls and set aside.

2. Place the broth, carrots, bouillon granules, and garlic in a 3-quart pot and bring to a boil. Drop the meatballs into the pot a few at a time until they have all been added. Cover and simmer over medium-low heat for 10 minutes. Use a slotted spoon to remove about half of the carrots. Place the carrots and about 1 cup of the broth in a blender and carefully blend at low speed until smooth. Pour the blended mixture back into the pot.

3. Add the escarole and orzo and simmer covered for an additional 9 minutes, or until the pasta is al dente. (Be careful not to overcook as the pasta will continue to cook a bit more in the hot soup.) Serve hot, topping each serving with a sprinkling of parsley and some grated Parmesan cheese if desired.

Nutritional Facts (per 1-cup serving)
CALORIES: 148 CARBOHYDRATES: 15 g
CHOLESTEROL: 24 mg FAT: 3.7 g SAT. FAT: 1.6 g
FIBER: 1.8 g PROTEIN: 13 g SODIUM: 358 mg
CALCIUM: 43 mg
   Diabetic exchanges: 1½ lean meat, ¾ starch, 1 vegetable

■ ■ ■

Southwestern Chicken Soup

YIELD: 7 SERVINGS

TORTILLA STRIPS
4 thin corn tortillas
Olive oil cooking spray
⅛ teaspoon salt

1 tablespoon extra virgin olive oil
1 medium yellow onion, chopped
1 teaspoon dried oregano
1 teaspoon ground cumin
3 cups water
14½-ounce can Mexican-style stewed tomatoes, puréed in a blender until smooth
½ cup diced carrot
2 teaspoons chicken bouillon granules
1¼ cups frozen whole kernel corn
1 cup diced zucchini squash
1½ cups shredded roasted skinless chicken

1. Preheat oven to 350°.

2. To make the tortilla strips, stack the tortillas on top of each other and cut them in half. Then cut each stack of halves into ½-inch wide strips. Coat a large nonstick baking sheet with the nonstick cooking spray and arrange the strips in a single layer on the sheet. Spray the tops of the strips lightly with the cooking spray and sprinkle with the salt. Bake for 10 to 12 minutes, until lightly browned and crisp. Set aside.

3. Place the olive oil in a 3-quart pot and place over medium heat. Add the onion, oregano, and cumin. Cover and cook for several minutes, until the onion starts to soften.

4. Add the water, blended tomatoes, carrot, and bouillon granules and bring to a boil. Reduce the heat to low, cover, and simmer for 15 minutes, until the carrots are tender. Add the corn and zucchini and simmer for 5 minutes more, until the zucchini are crisp-tender. Add the chicken and simmer for another minute or 2 to heat through. Serve hot, topping each serving with some of the tortilla strips.

Nutritional Facts (per 1-cup serving)
CALORIES: 137 CARBOHYDRATES: 12 g
CHOLESTEROL: 24 mg FAT: 3.7 g SAT. FAT: 0.7 g
FIBER: 2.2 g PROTEIN: 14 g SODIUM: 460 mg
CALCIUM: 41 mg
Diabetic exchanges: 1 lean meat, ½ starch, 1 vegetable

■ ■ ■

Chicken Tortellini Soup

YIELD: 8 SERVINGS

6 cups water
1 cup chopped onion
1 cup sliced carrots
½ cup sliced celery
1 tablespoon chicken bouillon granules
¾ teaspoon poultry seasoning
⅛ teaspoon ground black pepper
9 ounces (about 2½ cups) refrigerated cheese tortellini
1½ cups diced skinless roasted chicken
2 teaspoons dried parsley, finely crumbled

1. Combine the water, onion, carrots, celery, bouillon granules, poultry seasoning, and pepper in a 3-quart pot and bring to a boil. Reduce the heat to low, cover, and simmer for 15 minutes, until the vegetables are tender.

2. Using a slotted spoon, transfer half of the vegetables to a blender and pour in about 1 cup of the broth. Carefully blend at low speed to purée the vegetables. Return the blended mixture to the pot.

3. Add the tortellini to the pot and bring to a boil. Reduce the heat to medium-low, cover, and simmer for 5 minutes. Add the chicken and simmer covered for an additional 4 to 5 minutes, or until the tortellini is cooked through. Serve hot, topping each serving with a sprinkling of parsley.

Nutritional Facts (per 1-cup serving)
CALORIES: 159 CARBOHYDRATES: 18 g
CHOLESTEROL: 36 mg FAT: 3.8 g SAT. FAT: 1.6 g
FIBER: 1.7 g PROTEIN: 13 g SODIUM: 390 mg
CALCIUM: 74 mg
Diabetic exchanges: 1½ lean meat, 1 starch, ½ vegetable

■ ■ ■

Savory Chili

YIELD: 8 SERVINGS

1 pound 95% lean ground beef or turkey

1 cup chopped onion

1 cup grated carrots

½ cup finely chopped celery

14½-ounce can Mexican-style stewed tomatoes

2 cups tomato juice

2 tablespoons chili powder

1 teaspoon ground cumin

2 cans (15 ounces each) red kidney beans or
   pinto beans, or 1 can of each, drained

1. Coat a 3-quart pot with nonstick cooking spray and place over medium heat. Add the ground beef and cook, stirring to crumble, until the meat is no longer pink. Drain off and discard any fat. Add the onion, carrots, and celery to the pot. Cover and cook over medium heat for 5 to 7 minutes, until the vegetables soften.

2. Add the undrained tomatoes, tomato juice, chili powder, and cumin to the pot. Bring the mixture to a boil, reduce the heat to low, cover, and simmer, stirring occasionally, for 20 minutes. Add the beans and simmer covered for 10 minutes more.

3. Serve hot, topping each serving with some shredded reduced-fat cheddar or Monterey Jack cheese if desired.

Nutritional Facts (per 1-cup serving)
CALORIES: 232 CARBOHYDRATES: 31 g
CHOLESTEROL: 30 mg FAT: 3.4 g SAT. FAT: 1.1 g
FIBER: 11 g PROTEIN: 20 g SODIUM: 380 mg
CALCIUM: 38 mg
   Diabetic exchanges: 2½ lean meat, 1½ starch, 1½ vegetable

■ ■ ■

Cream of Asparagus Soup

YIELD: 4 SERVINGS

1 tablespoon margarine or butter

⅓ cup sliced scallions

1½ teaspoons crushed garlic

1½ cups chicken broth

3 cups 1-inch pieces fresh asparagus spears

¾ teaspoon fines herbes, herbes de Provence, or
   dried thyme

⅛ teaspoon salt

⅛ teaspoon ground white pepper

1½ cups nonfat or low-fat milk

2 tablespoons unbleached flour

1. Put the margarine or butter in a 2-quart nonstick pot and melt over medium heat. Add the scallions, cover, and cook for several minutes, until softened. Add the garlic and cook for about 10 seconds, just until the garlic begins to turn color and smell fragrant.

2. Add the broth, asparagus, herbs, salt, and white pepper and bring to a boil. Reduce

the heat to low, cover, and simmer for about 8 minutes, until the asparagus is tender. Pour the mixture into a blender and carefully blend at low speed to purée the asparagus. Return the mixture to the pot.

3. Place the milk and flour in the blender and blend to dissolve the flour. Add the milk mixture to the asparagus mixture. Increase the heat to medium and cook, stirring frequently, until the soup begins to boil. Cook, stirring constantly, for another minute or two, until the soup thickens slightly. Serve hot.

Nutritional Facts (per 1-cup serving)

CALORIES: 92 CARBOHYDRATES: 12 g CHOLESTEROL: 2 mg FAT: 2.6 g SAT. FAT: 0.7 g FIBER: 2.4 g PROTEIN: 6 g SODIUM: 386 mg CALCIUM: 140 mg

Diabetic exchanges: 1½ vegetable, ½ low-fat milk, ½ fat

■ ■ ■

Cream of Mushroom Soup

YIELD: 5 SERVINGS

1 tablespoon canola oil

1 cup chopped onion

2 teaspoons crushed garlic

4½ cups sliced fresh mushrooms

¾ teaspoon fines herbes or herbes de Provence

½ teaspoon salt

⅛ teaspoon ground white pepper

2 cups unsalted chicken broth

¼ cup medium-dry sherry

12-ounce can evaporated nonfat or low-fat milk

2 tablespoons cornstarch

1. Place the oil in a 2½ quart nonstick pot and preheat over medium heat. Add the onion, cover, and cook for several minutes, until the onion softens. Add the garlic, mushrooms, herbs, salt, and pepper and cook for several minutes, until the mushrooms soften and release their juices.

2. Add the broth and sherry and bring the mixture to a boil. Reduce the heat to low and cover and simmer for 10 minutes. Increase the heat to medium and add 1¼ cups of the evaporated milk. Cook, stirring frequently, until the milk just begins to boil.

3. Dissolve the cornstarch in the remaining evaporated milk and add it to the pot. Cook and stir for a couple of minutes, until the mixture boils and thickens slightly. Add another teaspoon or two of cornstarch if the mixture seems too thin (dissolve the cornstarch in an equal amount of milk or water before adding it to the pot). Serve hot.

Nutritional Facts (per 1-cup serving)

CALORIES: 125 CARBOHYDRATES: 16 g CHOLESTEROL: 2 mg FAT: 3.1 g SAT. FAT: 0.3 g FIBER: 1.5 g PROTEIN: 7 g SODIUM: 315 mg CALCIUM: 207 mg

Diabetic exchanges: 1 vegetable, ¼ starch, ½ low-fat milk, ½ fat

■ ■ ■

Tortellini Vegetable Soup

YIELD: 8 SERVINGS

¾ cup chopped onion

4 cups water

14½-ounce can diced tomatoes with
Italian seasonings

1 cup diced carrots

½ teaspoon salt

⅛ teaspoon ground black pepper

9 ounces (about 2½ cups) refrigerated cheese
tortellini

1 cup thinly sliced fresh mushrooms

1 cup zucchini, quartered lengthwise and
thinly sliced

1 cup (packed) chopped fresh spinach

2 teaspoons dried parsley, finely crumbled

1. Coat a 3-quart pot with nonstick cooking spray or 1 tablespoon of olive oil and add the onion. Cover and cook over medium heat for several minutes, until the onions start to soften.

2. Add the water, undrained tomatoes, carrots, salt, and pepper to the pot and bring to a boil. Reduce the heat to low, cover, and simmer for 15 minutes, until the carrots are tender.

3. Using a slotted spoon, transfer half of the vegetables to a blender and pour in about 1 cup of the liquid. Carefully blend at low speed to purée the vegetables. Return the blended mixture back to the pot.

4. Add the tortellini and mushrooms to the pot and bring to a boil. Reduce the heat to medium-low, cover, and cook for 5 minutes. Add the zucchini and cook covered for an additional 4 minutes. Add the spinach and cook for another minute, until the spinach wilts and the tortellini is cooked through. Serve hot, topping each serving with a sprinkling of parsley.

Nutritional Facts (per 1-cup serving)
CALORIES: 120 CARBOHYDRATES: 20 g
CHOLESTEROL: 12 mg FAT: 2.6 g SAT. FAT: 1.2 g
FIBER: 2.2 g PROTEIN: 5.2 g SODIUM: 368 mg
CALCIUM: 83 mg
    Diabetic exchanges: 1 starch, 1 vegetable, ½ fat

▪ ▪ ▪

Curried Butternut Squash Soup

YIELD: 7 SERVINGS

2 medium butternut squash (¾ pound each),
halved lengthwise and seeded

1½ tablespoons extra virgin olive oil

1 cup chopped onion

½ cup sliced celery

1 teaspoon crushed garlic

4 cups chicken or vegetable broth

2 medium Granny Smith apples, peeled
and chopped

1 teaspoon curry paste or curry powder

¼ teaspoon ground cinnamon

¼ teaspoon ground ginger

1. Preheat oven to 400°.

2. Coat a large baking sheet with nonstick cooking spray and lay the squash halves, cut sides down, on the sheets. Bake for about 45 minutes, until soft. Let the squash cool and scoop out the flesh. (There should be about 2 cups of squash.)

3. Place the olive oil in a 3-quart pot and add the onions, celery, and garlic. Cover and cook over medium heat for about 4 minutes, stirring several times, until the vegetables are soft.

4. Add half of the broth to the pot along with the apples and spices. Bring to a boil, then reduce the heat to low. Cover and simmer for 5 minutes, until the apples are soft.

5. Transfer the apple mixture and squash to a blender and carefully blend at low speed, leaving the lid slightly ajar (to allow steam to escape) until smooth. Pour the blended soup back into the pot and add the remaining broth. Cover and simmer for 5 additional minutes. Serve hot.

Nutritional Facts (per 1-cup serving)

CALORIES: 90 CARBOHYDRATES: 15 g CHOLESTEROL: 0 mg FAT: 3.5 g SAT. FAT: 0.4 g FIBER: 3.8 g PROTEIN: 1.2 g SODIUM: 398 mg CALCIUM: 49 mg

Diabetic exchanges: ½ starch, ½ fruit, ½ fat

▪ ▪ ▪

Garden Garbanzo Soup

YIELD: 4 SERVINGS

1 tablespoon extra virgin olive oil

½ cup chopped onion

1 can (15 ounces) garbanzo beans, drained

1 cup peeled and diced Yukon Gold potato (about 1 medium-large)

1 medium carrot, peeled and diced

2 to 3 teaspoons crushed garlic

1 bay leaf

2 cups reduced-sodium chicken or vegetable broth

1½ cups (moderately packed) chopped fresh spinach

1 teaspoon dried parsley or 1 tablespoon fresh

¼ cup grated Parmesan cheese (optional)

1. Coat a 2-quart pot with the olive oil and add the onions. Place the pot over medium heat, cover, and cook, stirring occasionally, for several minutes, until the onions soften.

2. Add the garbanzo beans, potato, carrot, garlic, bay leaf, and broth to the pot and bring to a boil. Reduce the heat to low, cover, and simmer for 20 minutes, until the vegetables are soft. Remove and discard the bay leaf.

3. Remove ¾ to 1 cup of the soup to a blender and process until smooth. Add the blended mixture back to the pot and then add the spinach and parsley. Bring the mixture to a boil, then reduce the heat to low, cover, and

simmer for 5 minutes, until the spinach is wilted and the flavors are well blended.

4. Serve hot, topping each serving with some of the Parmesan cheese, if desired.

Nutritional Facts (per 1-cup serving)

CALORIES: 175 CARBOHYDRATES: 27 g
CHOLESTEROL: 0 mg FAT: 5 g SAT. FAT: 0.6 g FIBER: 6.2 g
PROTEIN: 7 g SODIUM: 450 mg CALCIUM: 52 mg

Diabetic exchanges: 1 very lean meat, 1½ starch, 1 vegetable, 1 fat

▪ ▪ ▪

Lentil Soup with Spinach & Potatoes

YIELD: 8 SERVINGS

1 tablespoon extra virgin olive oil
1½ cups chopped onion
1¼ cups lentils
5 cups reduced-sodium chicken broth
1 tablespoon crushed garlic
1 teaspoon fines herbes or herbes de Provence
¼ teaspoon ground black pepper
2 cups diced Yukon gold potatoes
4 cups (moderately packed) chopped fresh spinach
⅓ cup grated Parmesan cheese

1. Coat the bottom of a 4-quart nonstick pot with the olive oil and place over medium heat. Add the onion, cover, and cook for several minutes, until the onion starts to soften.

2. Add the lentils, broth, garlic, herbs, and pepper to the pot and bring to a boil. Reduce the heat to low, cover, and simmer for 30 minutes. Add the potatoes and cook for an additional 20 minutes, until the lentils and potatoes are soft.

3. Add the spinach to the soup and cook for 3 to 5 minutes more, until the spinach wilts. Serve hot, topping each serving with some of the Parmesan cheese.

Nutritional Facts (per 1-cup serving)

CALORIES: 167 CARBOHYDRATES: 25 g
CHOLESTEROL: 3 mg FAT: 3.4 g SAT. FAT: 1.1 g
FIBER: 7 g PROTEIN: 10 g SODIUM: 492 mg
CALCIUM: 95 mg

Diabetic exchanges: 1 very lean meat, 1¼ starch, 1 vegetable, ½ fat

▪ ▪ ▪

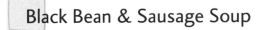

Black Bean & Sausage Soup

YIELD: 6 SERVINGS

8 ounces low-fat smoked sausage or kielbasa, sliced ¼-inch thick
¾ cup chopped Spanish onion
1 teaspoon crushed garlic
1 teaspoon ground cumin
1 teaspoon dried oregano
1¼ cups unsalted chicken broth
2 cans (15 ounces each) black beans, undrained
3 tablespoons finely chopped fresh cilantro or thinly sliced scallions

1. Coat a 2½-quart pot with nonstick cooking spray and add the sausage, onion, garlic, cumin, and oregano. Cover and cook over medium heat, stirring occasionally, for about 5 minutes, until the onions start to soften.

2. Add the broth to the pot. Place 1 cup of the beans in a shallow dish and mash with a fork. Add the mashed beans and the remaining beans to the pot. Bring to a boil and reduce the heat to low. Cover and simmer for 15 minutes, until the flavors are well blended. Serve hot, topping each serving with a sprinkling of cilantro or scallions. If desired, serve over brown rice.

—————————

Nutritional Facts (per 1-cup serving)
CALORIES: 182 CARBOHYDRATES: 25 g
CHOLESTEROL: 14 mg FAT: 2.5 g SAT. FAT: 0.5 g
FIBER: 8 g PROTEIN: 13 g SODIUM: 787 mg
CALCIUM: 65 mg
   Diabetic exchanges: 2½ lean meat, 1¼ starch, 1 vegetable

■ ■ ■

Butterbean Soup

YIELD: 10 SERVINGS

2 cups dried lima beans, cleaned and soaked
2 cups diced lean ham or 1 large meaty
   ham bone
1¼ cups chopped yellow onion
1 cup diced carrot

1 cup chopped celery (include some leaves)
6½ cups water
2 teaspoons dried sage
2 bay leaves
½ teaspoon salt
¼ teaspoon ground black pepper

1. Place all of the ingredients in a 4-quart pot and bring to a boil over high heat. Reduce the heat to low, cover, and simmer for about 2 hours, until the beans are soft and the liquid is thick. Add a little more water during cooking if the mixture becomes too dry.

2. If using a ham bone, remove the bone, trim off and dice the meat, and add it back to the soup. Serve hot.

—————————

Nutritional Facts (per 1-cup serving)
CALORIES: 180 CARBOHYDRATES: 30 g
CHOLESTEROL: 14 mg FAT: 1.1 g SAT. FAT: 0.4 g
FIBER: 9.3 g PROTEIN: 14 g SODIUM: 343 mg
CALCIUM: 45 mg
   Diabetic exchanges: 1 lean meat, 1½ starch, 1 vegetable

■ ■ ■

Turkey & Barley Soup

YIELD: 9 SERVINGS

1 tablespoon canola or extra virgin olive oil
2 cups sliced fresh mushrooms
1 medium yellow onion, chopped
1 cup chopped celery (include the leaves)

6 cups unsalted chicken broth

²/₃ cup hulled or pearl barley

1 tablespoon plus 1 teaspoon chicken
   bouillon granules

1½ teaspoons crushed garlic

1½ teaspoons fines herbes or dried thyme

1 teaspoon poultry seasoning

¼ teaspoon ground black pepper

1 cup sliced carrots

2 cups diced roasted skinless turkey or chicken

1. Place the oil in a 4-quart pot and preheat over medium heat. Add the mushrooms, onion, and celery and sauté for about 5 minutes, until tender.

2. Add the remaining ingredients, except for the carrots and turkey, and bring to a boil. Reduce the heat to low, cover, and simmer for 30 minutes.

3. Add the carrots and simmer covered for 30 minutes, until the carrots and barley are tender. Add the turkey and simmer for 5 minutes more. Serve hot.

Nutritional Facts (per 1-cup serving)
CALORIES: 149 CARBOHYDRATES: 15 g
CHOLESTEROL: 30 mg FAT: 2.6 g SAT. FAT: 0.4 g
FIBER: 3.2 g PROTEIN: 16 g SODIUM: 444 mg
CALCIUM: 36 mg
   Diabetic exchanges: 1 very lean meat, ¾ starch, ½ vegetable

▪ ▪ ▪

11. SENSATIONAL SALADS

Chockful of fresh produce, salads play a key role in promoting excellent health. Leafy greens and most fresh raw vegetables are very low in calories and carbohydrate, so they help keep blood sugar levels under control. Other salad ingredients, like skinless poultry, seafood, whole grains, pasta, legumes, and fruits, offer their own unique nutritional benefits.

Besides being supernutritious, salads are among the most versatile of dishes. Depending on their ingredients, they can be a protein-packed entrée or a refreshing side dish. Many salads can also be made ahead of time, making them a natural for entertaining, picnics, and potluck dinners.

If you are watching your weight, beware that all salads are not created equal. Salads made with high-fat meats and cheeses drenched in full-fat mayo or oily dressings can bust your calorie budget in a hurry. Rest assured that the recipes in this chapter will help you maintain your light and healthy lifestyle. Ingredients like lean meats; low-fat cheeses; and light mayo, sour cream, and dressings are combined with crisp vegetables, ripe fruits, satisfying pastas, and nutritious whole-grains, and legumes to create an array of sensational salads that are sure to make any meal special.

West Coast Cobb Salad

YIELD: 4 SERVINGS

12 cups torn romaine lettuce

2 cups diced grilled chicken breast or roast turkey

1 cup diced tomato

1 cup diced avocado

1 medium carrot, shredded with a potato peeler

½ cup chopped red onion

2 hard boiled eggs, chopped

4 slices turkey bacon, cooked and crumbled

¾ cup shredded nonfat or reduced-fat Monterey
    Jack cheese

¼ cup chopped walnuts

¾ cup nonfat or light ranch or olive oil
    vinaigrette salad dressing

1. Arrange a quarter of the salad greens over the bottoms of each of 4 plates. Top the lettuce on each plate with a quarter of the chicken or turkey and a quarter of the tomato, avocado, carrot, and onion.

2. Sprinkle each salad with some of the egg, bacon, cheese, and walnuts. Serve immediately accompanied by the dressing.

Nutritional Facts (per serving)
CALORIES: 413 CARBOHYDRATES: 27 g
CHOLESTEROL: 166 mg FAT: 16 g SAT. FAT: 2.7 g FIBER: 7 g
PROTEIN: 40 g SODIUM: 838 mg CALCIUM: 243 mg
    Diabetic exchanges: 4 lean meat, 4 vegetable, 2 fat

■ ■ ■

Southwestern Chicken Caesar Salad

YIELD: 4 SERVINGS

DRESSING

¼ cup plus 2 tablespoons nonfat or low-
    fat mayonnaise

2 tablespoons extra virgin olive oil

1½ teaspoons lemon juice

1 teaspoon crushed garlic

1 to 1½ teaspoons chopped chipotle peppers
    in adobo sauce*

10 cups torn romaine lettuce

2 cups diced grilled chicken

16 grape tomatoes

½ cup frozen corn, thawed and drained

½ cup black beans, rinsed and drained

½ cup grated Parmesan cheese

1. To make the dressing, combine all of the ingredients in a mini blender jar and blend to mix well. Set aside.

2. Place the lettuce, chicken, tomatoes, corn, and black beans in a large bowl and toss to mix well. Add the dressing and toss to mix. Add the Parmesan cheese and toss again. Divide the mixture between 4 serving plates and serve immediately.

Nutritional Facts (per serving)

CALORIES: 317 CARBOHYDRATES: 19 g
CHOLESTEROL: 72 mg FAT: 14 g SAT. FAT: 4.8 g FIBER: 5 g
PROTEIN: 30 g SODIUM: 613 mg CALCIUM: 247 mg

   Diabetic exchanges: 3 lean meat, 3 vegetable,
1½ fat

*Chipotle peppers in adobo sauce are smoked red jalapeño peppers that are canned in a tomato-vinegar sauce. Small cans can be found in the Mexican section of most grocery stores. Be sure to wear gloves when working with all hot peppers, as the hot components can cause a burning sensation. Leftovers can be frozen in ice cube trays and transferred to freezer bags for later use.

■ ■ ■

Chicken Taco Salad

YIELD: 5 SERVINGS

FILLING

15-ounce can chili beans, undrained

¾ cup chunky-style salsa

1 tablespoon chili powder

2 cups diced or shredded roasted chicken

12 cups torn romaine lettuce

¾ cup chopped tomatoes

¾ cup shredded nonfat or reduced-fat Monterey
   Jack or Mexican blend cheese

½ cup nonfat or light sour cream

⅓ cup sliced black olives

1 medium avocado, peeled and sliced

2 ounces low-fat tortilla chips (about
   25 chips)

1. To make the filling, place the beans, salsa, and chili powder in a 2-quart nonstick pot. Cover and bring the mixture to a boil. Add the chicken and cook for another minute to heat through. Remove the pot from the heat and set aside to keep warm.

2. To assemble the salad, arrange a fifth of the lettuce over the bottom of each of 5 large plates and top with about ⅞ cup of the filling. Garnish each salad with some of the tomatoes, cheese, sour cream, olives, and avocado slices. Arrange a fifth of the chips around the outer edges of each plate and serve immediately.

Nutritional Facts (per serving)

CALORIES: 353 CARBOHYDRATES: 37 g
CHOLESTEROL: 52 mg FAT: 11 g SAT. FAT: 2 g FIBER: 9 g
PROTEIN: 29 g SODIUM: 966 mg CALCIUM: 230 mg

   Diabetic exchanges: 3½ very lean meat, 1½ starch,
3 vegetable, 1½ fat

■ ■ ■

Greek Chicken Chop Salad

YIELD: 4 SERVINGS

10 cups chopped romaine lettuce

1 cup diced plum tomatoes

1 cup diced seeded cucumber or coarsely
   chopped marinated artichoke hearts

2 cups diced grilled chicken breast

½ cup chopped red onion

¼ cup finely chopped fresh parsley

½ cup crumbled reduced-fat feta cheese

¾ cup canned garbanzo beans, rinsed and
  drained
¼ cup sliced black olives
½ cup light olive oil vinaigrette salad dressing

1. Layer all of the ingredients except for
the salad dressing in a large bowl.

2. Pour the dressing over the top and toss
to mix well. Serve immediately.

Nutritional Facts (per serving)
CALORIES: 321 CARBOHYDRATES: 20 g
CHOLESTEROL: 52 mg FAT: 15 g SAT. FAT: 2.9 g
FIBER: 5.5 g PROTEIN: 28 g SODIUM: 721 mg
CALCIUM: 137 mg
   Diabetic exchanges: 3½ very lean meat, 3½ veg-
etable, 2 fat

■ ■ ■

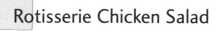

Rotisserie Chicken Salad

YIELD: 4 SERVINGS

10 cups torn romaine lettuce or mixed
  salad greens
¾ cup coarsely shredded red cabbage
1 medium carrot, shredded with a potato peeler
4 thin slices red onion, separated into rings
2 cups skinless diced rotisserie chicken
12 cherry or grape tomatoes
½ cup shredded nonfat or reduced-fat cheddar
  or Monterey Jack cheese
3 slices turkey bacon, cooked, drained, and
  crumbled

¼ cup dark raisins
¼ cup chopped walnuts
½ cup Buttermilk-Herb Dressing (recipe follows)
  or nonfat or light ranch salad dressing

1. Combine the lettuce, cabbage, carrot,
and onion in a large bowl and toss to mix
well. Arrange a quarter of the lettuce mixture
over the bottoms of each of 4 plates. Top the
lettuce on each plate with a quarter of the
chicken and arrange 4 of the tomatoes around
the outer edges of each plate.

2. Sprinkle each salad with some of the
cheese, bacon, raisins, and walnuts. Serve immediately accompanied by the dressing.

Nutritional Facts (per serving)
CALORIES: 355 CARBOHYDRATES: 19 g
CHOLESTEROL: 73 mg FAT: 17 g SAT. FAT: 2 g FIBER: 4.3 g
PROTEIN: 32 g SODIUM: 439 mg CALCIUM: 192 mg
   Diabetic exchanges: 3½ lean meat, 3½ vegetable,
3 fat

■ ■ ■

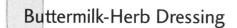

Buttermilk-Herb Dressing

YIELD: 1 CUP

⅓ cup nonfat or low-fat buttermilk
⅓ cup nonfat or light mayonnaise
¼ cup extra virgin olive oil or canola oil
2 teaspoons white wine vinegar
1 teaspoon Dijon mustard
1 teaspoon crushed garlic

½ teaspoon dried parsley

¼ teaspoon dried dill

⅛ teaspoon ground black pepper

1. Combine all of the ingredients in a mini blender jar and blend to mix well.

2. Serve immediately or cover and refrigerate until ready to use.

Nutritional Facts (per tablespoon)

CALORIES: 35 CARBOHYDRATES: 1 g CHOLESTEROL: 0 mg FAT: 3.4 g SAT. FAT: 0.5 g FIBER: 0 g PROTEIN: 0.2 g SODIUM: 48 mg CALCIUM: 7 mg

Diabetic exchanges: ½ fat

■ ■ ■

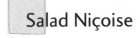

Salad Niçoise

YIELD: 4 SERVINGS

8 ounces small new potatoes, halved

2½ cups cut fresh green beans

½ cup light olive oil vinaigrette salad dressing

8 cups torn romaine, Boston, or bibb lettuce

4 slices red onion, separated into rings

12-ounce can albacore tuna in water, drained

4 hard-boiled eggs, peeled and quartered

16 cherry or grape tomatoes

¼ cup sliced black olives

1. Place the potatoes in a 2-quart pot and cover with water. Boil for about 12 minutes, until tender. Remove the potatoes with a slotted spoon, rinse with cool water, and set aside. Add the green beans to the pot and boil for about 3 minutes, until crisp-tender. Rinse the beans with cool water and drain well. (You can cook the potatoes and beans the day before and refrigerate until ready to assemble the salads.)

2. When ready to assemble the salads, slice the potatoes ¼-inch thick and place in a bowl with the green beans. Add ¼ cup of the salad dressing and toss to mix. Set aside.

3. Arrange a quarter of the lettuce over the bottom of each of four serving plates and top with a quarter of the onion rings. Arrange a quarter of the tuna and four egg quarters in the center of each salad and drizzle each salad with a tablespoon of the remaining dressing. Arrange a quarter of the potato mixture and 4 tomatoes around the outer edges of each plate and top with a sprinkling of olives. Serve immediately.

Nutritional Facts (per serving)

CALORIES: 347 CARBOHYDRATES: 29 g CHOLESTEROL: 214 mg FAT: 12 g SAT. FAT: 1.4 g FIBER: 5.2 g PROTEIN: 37 g SODIUM: 680 mg CALCIUM: 116 mg

Diabetic exchanges: 3 very lean meat, 3 vegetable, 1 starch, 2 fat

■ ■ ■

Asian Chicken Chop Salad

YIELD: 4 SERVINGS

10 cups coarsely chopped romaine lettuce or
    mixed salad greens
1 cup coarsely shredded purple cabbage
¾ cup small broccoli florets
8-ounce can pineapple chunks in juice, well
    drained
½ cup sliced canned water chestnuts, drained
    and coarsely chopped
½ cup diced red bell pepper
2½ cups diced grilled or roasted chicken
½ cup sliced scallions
½ cup Soy-Sesame Dressing (below)

1. Layer all of the ingredients except for
the salad dressing in a large bowl.

2. Pour the dressing over the top and toss
to mix well. Serve immediately.

Nutritional Facts (per serving)
CALORIES: 311 CARBOHYDRATES: 22 g
CHOLESTEROL: 75 mg FAT: 11.5 g SAT. FAT: 1.6 g
FIBER: 6 g PROTEIN: 31 g SODIUM: 344 mg
CALCIUM: 98 mg
    Diabetic exchanges: 3 lean meat, 3 vegetable,
½ fruit, 2 fat

■ ■ ■

Soy-Sesame Dressing

YIELD: ⅞ CUP

¼ cup light (reduced-sugar) apricot fruit spread
¼ cup rice vinegar
¼ cup dark roasted sesame oil
2 tablespoons reduced-sodium soy sauce
½ teaspoon ground ginger

1. Combine all of the ingredients in a
blender and blend until smooth.

2. Serve immediately or cover and refrigerate until ready to use. Shake well before serving.

Nutritional Facts (per tablespoon)
CALORIES: 40 CARBOHYDRATES: 1.7 g
CHOLESTEROL: 0 mg FAT: 3.9 g SAT. FAT: 0.6 g FIBER: 0 g
PROTEIN: 0 g SODIUM: 128 mg CALCIUM: 0 mg
    Diabetic exchanges: 1 fat

Artichoke Chicken Salad

YIELD: 4 SERVINGS

1½ cups shredded roasted chicken breast
1 cup marinated artichoke hearts, drained and
    coarsely chopped
½ cup 1-inch pieces roasted or broiled
    asparagus spears (page 169)
¼ cup chopped roasted red bell pepper

3 to 4 tablespoons light olive oil vinaigrette or
Italian salad dressing

1/8 teaspoon coarsely ground black pepper

1. Combine the chicken, artichoke hearts, asparagus, and bell pepper in a medium bowl and toss to mix well. Add the salad dressing and pepper and toss again.

2. Let the salad sit for 15 minutes before serving or cover and chill until ready to serve. If desired, serve on a bed of fresh salad greens garnished with a sprinkling of blue cheese crumbles and chopped walnuts, or serve in lettuce-lined pita pockets.

Nutritional Facts (per ¾-cup serving)
CALORIES: 148 CARBOHYDRATES: 5 g
CHOLESTEROL: 45 mg FAT: 5.1 g SAT. FAT: 1.5 g
FIBER: 2 g PROTEIN: 18 g SODIUM: 301 mg
CALCIUM: 20 mg
Diabetic exchanges: 2 very lean meat, 1 vegetable, 1 fat

■ ■ ■

Cranberry-Crunch Chicken Salad

YIELD: 6 SERVINGS

3 cups diced roasted chicken or turkey

2 cups cooked wild rice

2 cups peeled chopped Granny Smith apples
(about 2½ medium)

1 cup thinly sliced celery

½ cup dried sweetened cranberries

½ cup chopped walnuts or toasted pecans
(p. 233)

1 cup nonfat or light mayonnaise

1. Place the chicken or turkey, wild rice, apples, celery, cranberries, and nuts in a large bowl and toss to mix well. Add the mayonnaise and toss to mix well, adding a little more mayonnaise if the mixture seems too dry. Cover the salad and refrigerate for at least 2 hours before serving. Serve over a bed of fresh salad greens or mound each serving into the center of a cantaloupe half if desired.

Nutritional Facts (per 1½-cup serving)
CALORIES: 286 CARBOHYDRATES: 24 g
CHOLESTEROL: 60 mg FAT: 8.8 g SAT. FAT: 1.1 g
FIBER: 2.8 g PROTEIN: 27 g SODIUM: 351 mg
CALCIUM: 29 mg
Diabetic exchanges: 2½ very lean meat, ½ starch, 1 fruit, 1 fat

■ ■ ■

Artichoke & Sun-Dried Tomato Tuna Salad

YIELD: 4 SERVINGS

12-ounce can albacore tuna in water, drained

1½ cups marinated artichoke hearts, drained
(reserve the marinade)

¼ to ⅓ cup chopped sun-dried tomatoes packed
in olive oil, undrained

1 ½ tablespoons finely chopped fresh basil or
1 ½ teaspoons dried
¼ teaspoon coarsely ground black pepper

1. Place the tuna, artichoke hearts, sun-dried tomatoes, basil, and pepper in a medium-sized bowl. Add a couple of tablespoons of the reserved artichoke marinade and toss to mix well. Add a little more marinade if the mixture seems too dry.

2. Serve immediately or cover and chill until ready to serve. If desired, serve on a bed of fresh salad greens, in whole-wheat pita pockets, or whole-wheat wraps lined with mixed salad greens.

Nutritional Facts (per ¾-cup serving)
CALORIES: 155 CARBOHYDRATES: 5 g
CHOLESTEROL: 36 mg FAT: 5 g SAT. FAT: 0.4 g
FIBER: 4.1 g PROTEIN: 24 g SODIUM: 447 mg
CALCIUM: 40 mg
Diabetic exchanges: 2½ very lean meat,
1 vegetable, 1 fat

▪ ▪ ▪

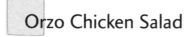

Orzo Chicken Salad

For variety, substitute canned tuna for the chicken.

YIELD: 6 SERVINGS

1 cup orzo pasta
2 cups diced roasted chicken breast

¾ cup frozen (thawed) green peas
½ cup sliced scallions
½ cup crumbled reduced-fat feta cheese
⅓ cup sun-dried tomatoes packed in olive oil, drained and chopped (reserve the oil)
2 tablespoons finely chopped fresh dill or
2 teaspoons dried

DRESSING
2 tablespoons oil from the sun-dried tomatoes
2 tablespoons lemon juice
1 teaspoon crushed garlic
½ teaspoon salt
¼ teaspoon ground black pepper

1. Cook the orzo according to package directions. Drain, rinse with cool water, and drain again. Place the orzo, chicken, peas, scallions, feta, tomatoes, and dill in a large bowl and toss to mix.

2. To make the dressing, place all of the dressing ingredients in a small bowl and stir to mix well. Pour the dressing over the orzo mixture and toss to mix. Cover and refrigerate for at least 1 hour before serving. Serve over a bed of fresh salad greens if desired.

Nutritional Facts (per 1⅛-cup serving)
CALORIES: 274 CARBOHYDRATES: 26 g
CHOLESTEROL: 43 mg FAT: 8.8 g SAT. FAT: 2.1 g
FIBER: 2.1 g PROTEIN: 22 g SODIUM: 398 mg
CALCIUM: 59 mg
Diabetic exchanges: 2 lean meat, 1½ starch, ½ vegetable, 1 fat

▪ ▪ ▪

Peanutty Shrimp & Noodle Salad

YIELD: 6 SERVINGS

8 ounces udon noodles

2 cups small broccoli florets

2½ cups cooked peeled and deveined shrimp

¾ cup matchstick-sized pieces red bell pepper

½ cup sliced scallions

8-ounce can bamboo shoots, drained

¼ cup chopped roasted peanuts

DRESSING

¼ cup rice vinegar

2 tablespoons reduced-sodium soy sauce

2 tablespoons peanut butter

1½ tablespoons honey

1 tablespoon sesame oil

1 teaspoon crushed garlic

¾ teaspoon ground ginger

1. Cook the noodles until almost al dente. About 1 minute before the noodles are done, add the broccoli and cook until crisp-tender. Drain, rinse with cold water, and drain again. Transfer to a large bowl.

2. Add the shrimp, red bell pepper, scallions and bamboo shoots to the pasta mixture.

3. Combine all of the dressing ingredients in a blender and blend until smooth. Pour over the pasta mixture and toss to mix well. Cover and chill before serving.

4. If desired, serve the salad over a bed of fresh spinach or salad greens. Top each serving with a sprinkling of the peanuts.

Nutritional Facts (per 1½-cup serving)
CALORIES: 313 CARBOHYDRATES: 36 g
CHOLESTEROL: 115 mg FAT: 9.6 g SAT. FAT: 1.5 g
FIBER: 4.5 g PROTEIN: 22 g SODIUM: 545 mg
CALCIUM: 64 mg
    Diabetic exchanges: 2 very lean meat, 2 starch, 1 vegetable, 1½ fat

■ ■ ■

Curried Orzo & Vegetable Salad

YIELD: 8 SERVINGS

1 cup uncooked orzo pasta

1½ cups small broccoli florets

1½ cups small cauliflower florets

⅓ cup dark or golden raisins

⅓ cup chopped roasted salted peanuts

DRESSING

½ cup plus 2 tablespoons nonfat or light
    mayonnaise

1 to 2 teaspoons mild curry paste

1. Cook the orzo al dente according to package directions. One minute before the orzo is done, add the broccoli and cauliflower to the pot and cook for 1 minute, until the broccoli turns bright green and the vegetables

are crisp-tender. Drain the orzo and vegetables, rinse with cool water, and drain again.

2. Place the orzo mixture in a large bowl, add the raisins and peanuts, and toss to mix well. To make the dressing, place the mayonnaise and curry paste in a small bowl and stir to mix well. Add the dressing to the salad and toss to mix well.

3. Cover the salad and chill for at least 2 hours before serving. Mix in a little more mayonnaise just before serving if the salad seems too dry.

_____

Nutritional Facts (per ¾-cup serving)
CALORIES: 155 CARBOHYDRATES: 25 g CHOLESTEROL: 0 mg
FAT: 3.5 g SAT. FAT: 0.4 g FIBER: 2.4 g PROTEIN: 5.3 g
SODIUM: 162 mg CALCIUM: 21 mg
    Diabetic exchanges: 1¼ starch, 1 vegetable, ½ fat

■ ■ ■

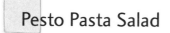

Pesto Pasta Salad

YIELD: 8 SERVINGS

8 ounces penne pasta
1½ cups small grape tomatoes

PESTO
¾ cup packed fresh spinach leaves
¾ cup packed fresh basil leaves
3 tablespoons extra virgin olive oil
⅓ cup grated Parmesan cheese
¼ teaspoon salt
¼ teaspoon ground black pepper

1. Cook the pasta al dente according to package directions. Drain, rinse with cool water, and drain again.

2. Place all of the pesto ingredients in a food processor and process into a paste. Add the pesto and tomatoes to the pasta and toss to mix well. Cover and chill for at least 1 hour before serving.

_____

Nutritional Facts (per ¾-cup serving)
CALORIES: 178 CARBOHYDRATES: 23 g CHOLESTEROL: 3 mg
FAT: 6.8 g SAT. FAT: 1.6 g FIBER: 1.3 g PROTEIN: 6 g
SODIUM: 158 mg CALCIUM: 78 mg
    Diabetic exchanges: 1¼ starch, ½ vegetable, 1 fat

■ ■ ■

Tabbouleh Fruit Salad

YIELD: 6 SERVINGS

2½ cups prepared bulgur wheat
¾ cup seedless red grapes
½ cup chopped dried apricots
½ cup sliced scallions
¼ cup plus 2 tablespoons sliced almonds or
   pine nuts
¼ cup finely chopped fresh parsley
2 tablespoons finely chopped fresh mint

DRESSING
2 tablespoons extra virgin olive oil
2 tablespoons lemon juice
½ teaspoon salt
⅛ teaspoon ground black pepper

1. Combine the bulgur wheat, grapes, apricots, scallions, almonds or pine nuts, parsley, and mint and toss to mix well. Combine the dressing ingredients in a small bowl and stir to mix well. Add the dressing to the salad and toss to mix well.

2. Cover the salad and chill for at least 1 hour before serving.

***

Nutritional Facts (per ¾-cup serving)
CALORIES: 186 CARBOHYDRATES: 27 g
CHOLESTEROL: 0 mg FAT: 8.2 g SAT. FAT: 0.9 g
FIBER: 5.7 g PROTEIN: 4.6 g SODIUM: 204 mg
CALCIUM: 42 mg
  Diabetic exchanges: 1 starch, 1 fruit, 1 fat

■ ■ ■

Spinach & Mushroom Salad

YIELD: 4 SERVINGS

6 cups fresh spinach leaves
1 cup sliced fresh mushrooms
2 slices red or sweet white onion, separated
  into rings
¼ cup shredded carrot
2 hard-boiled eggs, chopped
2 slices turkey bacon, cooked, drained, and
  crumbled
¼ cup shredded nonfat or reduced-fat
  cheddar cheese
½ cup Buttermilk-Herb Dressing (p. 155) or
  light ranch dressing

1. Combine the spinach, mushrooms, onion, and carrot in a large bowl and toss to mix.

2. Place a quarter of the salad mixture on each of 4 salad plates and top each salad with some of the eggs, bacon, and cheese. Serve immediately accompanied by the dressing.

***

Nutritional Facts (per serving)
CALORIES: 134 CARBOHYDRATES: 7 g
CHOLESTEROL: 95 mg FAT: 8.9 g SAT. FAT: 1 g
FIBER: 1.5 g PROTEIN: 6.5 g SODIUM: 221 mg
CALCIUM: 107 mg
  Diabetic exchanges: 1½ vegetable, 1 lean meat, 1 fat

■ ■ ■

Orange-Onion Salad

YIELD: 4 SERVINGS

6 cups prewashed mixed baby salad greens
1 cup fresh orange segments or 1 can
  (11-ounces) mandarin orange in juice, drained
2 slices red onion, separated into rings
¼ cup pine nuts or chopped walnuts
¼ cup Citrus Vinaigrette (below) or light
  balsamic vinaigrette salad dressing

1. Place 1½ cups of the salad greens on each of 4 serving plates. Top the greens on each plate with a quarter of the orange sections, a few onion rings, and a sprinkling of walnuts or pine nuts.

2. Drizzle some of the dressing over each salad and serve immediately.

Nutritional Facts (per serving)
CALORIES: 154 CARBOHYDRATES: 14 g
CHOLESTEROL: 0 mg FAT: 10.6 g SAT. FAT: 0.7 g
FIBER: 3.6 g PROTEIN: 3.9 g SODIUM: 152 mg
CALCIUM: 60 mg
    Diabetic exchanges: 1 vegetable, ½ fruit, 2 fat

■ ■ ■

Citrus Vinaigrette

YIELD: ABOUT ½ CUP

¼ cup extra virgin olive oil
2 tablespoons white wine vinegar
1 tablespoon lemon juice
1 tablespoon frozen (thawed) orange juice concentrate
1 tablespoon honey
½ teaspoon salt
¼ teaspoon dried thyme
¼ teaspoon ground black pepper

1. Combine all of the ingredients in a blender and blend for 1 minute to mix well.

2. Serve immediately or cover and refrigerate until ready to use. Shake well before serving.

Nutritional Facts (per tablespoon)
CALORIES: 64 CARBOHYDRATES: 2.8 g
CHOLESTEROL: 0 mg FAT: 6 g SAT. FAT: 0.8 g

FIBER: 0 g PROTEIN: 0 g SODIUM: 130 mg
CALCIUM: 2 mg
    Diabetic exchanges: 1 fat

■ ■ ■

Light Carrot-Raisin Salad

YIELD: 8 SERVINGS

3 cups coarsely shredded carrots
1 cup diced unpeeled Gala or Empire apple
½ cup thinly sliced celery
½ cup dark raisins

DRESSING
½ cup nonfat or light mayonnaise
¼ cup nonfat or light sour cream
1 tablespoon sugar substitute or sugar

1. Place the carrots, apple, celery, and raisins in a medium bowl and toss to mix.

2. Combine the dressing ingredients in a small bowl and stir to mix well. Add the dressing to the salad and toss to mix. Serve immediately or cover and refrigerate for several hours before serving.

Nutritional Facts (per ⅔-cup serving)
CALORIES: 68 CARBOHYDRATES: 16 g CHOLESTEROL: 0 mg
FAT: 0.2 g SAT. FAT: 0 g FIBER: 1.8 g PROTEIN: 1.2 g
SODIUM: 129 mg CALCIUM: 26 mg
    Diabetic exchanges: 1 vegetable, ¾ fruit

■ ■ ■

Cilantro-Carrot Salad

YIELD: 4 SERVINGS

2 cups coarsely shredded carrots
3 tablespoons finely chopped fresh cilantro

DRESSING
1 tablespoon olive or canola oil
1 tablespoon lime juice
1 teaspoon honey
⅛ teaspoon salt

1. Combine the carrots and cilantro in a medium bowl and toss to mix well.

2. Combine the oil, lime juice, honey, and salt in a small bowl and stir to mix well. Pour the dressing over the salad and toss to mix well. Serve immediately or cover and refrigerate until ready to serve.

Nutritional Facts (per ½-cup serving)
CALORIES: 60 CARBOHYDRATES: 7 g CHOLESTEROL: 0 mg FAT: 3.5 g SAT. FAT: 0.5 mg FIBER: 1.7 g PROTEIN: 0.6 g SODIUM: 185 mg CALCIUM: 17 mg
   Diabetic exchanges: 1 vegetable, ½ fat

■ ■ ■

Summer Tomato Salad

YIELD: 4 SERVINGS

4 large plum tomatoes, sliced
½ medium red or sweet white onion, thinly sliced and separated into rings

¼ cup chopped fresh basil
3 tablespoons light olive oil vinaigrette salad dressing

1. Combine the tomatoes, onion rings, and basil in a medium bowl and toss to mix well. Pour the dressing over the salad and toss again.

2. Let the mixture sit at room temperature for 15 to 30 minutes before serving.

Nutritional Facts (per serving)
CALORIES: 45 CARBOHYDRATES: 6 g CHOLESTEROL: 0 mg FAT: 2.5 g SAT. FAT: 0.4 g FIBER: 1.2 g PROTEIN: 0.9 g SODIUM: 97 mg CALCIUM: 11 mg
   Diabetic exchanges: 1 vegetable, ½ fat

■ ■ ■

Asian-style Cole Slaw

YIELD: 8 SERVINGS

4 cups coarsely shredded green cabbage
1½ cups coarsely shredded purple cabbage
1 small yellow bell pepper, cut into matchstick-sized pieces
½ cup coarsely shredded carrot
½ cup thinly sliced scallions
⅓ to ½ cup chopped fresh cilantro

DRESSING
¼ cup rice vinegar
3 tablespoons peanut butter
2 tablespoons canola oil
1½ tablespoons reduced-sodium soy sauce

1 ½ tablespoons honey

1 teaspoon ground ginger

1. Combine the cabbages, bell pepper, carrot, scallions, and cilantro in a bowl and toss to mix.

2. Combine all of the dressing ingredients in a small bowl and whisk until smooth. Pour over the cabbage mixture and toss to mix well. Serve immediately or cover and refrigerate until ready to serve.

Nutritional Facts (per ⅔-cup serving)

CALORIES: 90 CARBOHYDRATES: 7 g CHOLESTEROL: 0 mg
FAT: 6.5 g SAT. FAT: 0.7 g FIBER: 1.7 g PROTEIN: 2 g
SODIUM: 308 mg CALCIUM: 21 mg
    Diabetic exchanges: 1½ vegetable, 1 fat

■ ■ ■

Cranberry-Apple Spinach Salad

YIELD: 4 SERVINGS

6 cups moderately packed fresh spinach
    leaves

¼ cup light balsamic vinaigrette salad dressing or
    Citrus Vinaigrette (p. 163)

1 cup matchstick-sized pieces apple

¼ cup dried cranberries

¼ cup chopped walnuts or toasted pecans
    (p. 233)

¼ cup crumbled reduced-fat feta or
    blue cheese

1. Place the spinach leaves and salad dressing in a large bowl and toss to mix well. Divide the mixture between 4 salad plates.

2. Top the spinach on each plate with a quarter of the apples, cranberries, nuts, and cheese. Serve immediately.

Nutritional Facts (per serving)

CALORIES: 141 CARBOHYDRATES: 13 g
CHOLESTEROL: 2 mg FAT: 8.3 g SAT. FAT: 1 g FIBER: 2 g
PROTEIN: 4.7 g SODIUM: 272 mg CALCIUM: 69 mg
    Diabetic exchanges: 1 vegetable, ½ fruit, 1½ fat

■ ■ ■

Mediterranean White Bean Salad

YIELD: 6 SERVINGS

15-ounce can white beans, rinsed and drained

¾ cup chopped seeded plum tomato (about
    3 medium)

¾ cup diced peeled and seeded cucumber
    (about 1 medium)

⅓ cup sliced scallions

½ cup finely chopped fresh parsley

¼ cup light olive oil vinaigrette salad dressing

1 teaspoon crushed garlic

¼ teaspoon coarsely ground black pepper

1. Combine the beans, tomato, cucumber, scallions, and parsley in a large bowl.

2. Add the salad dressing, garlic, and pepper and toss gently to mix. Cover the salad

and refrigerate for at least 1 hour before serving.

Nutritional Facts (per ½-cup serving)

CALORIES: 76 CARBOHYDRATES: 15 g CHOLESTEROL: 0 mg FAT: 2.4 g SAT. FAT: 0.2 g FIBER: 4.1 g PROTEIN: 4.6 g SODIUM: 304 mg CALCIUM: 49 mg

Diabetic exchanges: ½ very lean meat, ½ starch, 1 vegetable, ½ fat

■ ■ ■

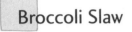

Crunchy Cabbage Salad

YIELD: 8 SERVINGS

5 cups coarsely shredded cabbage

1-pound can pineapple tidbits in juice, well drained

8-ounce can water chestnuts, drained and chopped

½ cup shredded reduced-fat cheddar cheese

⅓ cup chopped toasted pecans (p. 233)

½ cup nonfat or light mayonnaise

¼ cup light sour cream

1. Place all of the ingredients except for the mayonnaise and sour cream in a large bowl and toss to mix.

2. Combine the mayonnaise and sour cream, add to the cabbage mixture, and toss to mix well. Cover the salad and refrigerate for at least 1 hour before serving.

Nutritional Facts (per ⅔-cup serving)

CALORIES: 124 CARBOHYDRATES: 15 g CHOLESTEROL: 6 mg FAT: 5.4 g SAT. FAT: 1.3 g

FIBER: 2.9 g PROTEIN: 4.2 g SODIUM: 167 mg CALCIUM: 104 mg

Diabetic exchanges: 1 vegetable, ½ fruit, 1 fat

■ ■ ■

Broccoli Slaw

YIELD: 8 SERVINGS

12-ounce package broccoli slaw mix (about 5 cups)

1 medium apple, cut into matchstick-sized pieces

⅓ cup dark raisins

⅓ cup roasted salted sunflower seeds

DRESSING

½ cup plus 2 tablespoons nonfat or light mayonnaise

1 tablespoon sugar substitute or sugar

1 tablespoon apple cider vinegar

1. Combine the broccoli, apple, raisins, and sunflower seeds in a large bowl and toss to mix well.

2. Combine the dressing ingredients in a small bowl and stir to mix well. Add the dressing to the broccoli mixture and toss to mix well. Add a little more mayonnaise if the salad seems too dry.

3. Cover the salad and chill for at least 1 hour before serving.

Nutritional Facts (per ¾-cup serving)

CALORIES: 80 CARBOHYDRATES: 13 g CHOLESTEROL: 0 mg FAT: 2.7 g SAT. FAT: 0.3 g FIBER: 2.7 g PROTEIN: 2.2 g SODIUM: 186 mg CALCIUM: 26 mg

Diabetic exchanges: 1 vegetable, ½ fruit, ½ fat

■ ■ ■

Cool Mandarin-Pineapple Salad

YIELD: 8 SERVINGS

8-ounce can crushed pineapple in juice

1 package (4-serving size) sugar-free lime or orange gelatin

1 ½ cups nonfat or light cottage cheese

1 10-ounce can mandarin oranges in juice, drained

½ cup chopped toasted pecans (p. 233)

1 ½ to 2 cups nonfat or light whipped topping

1. Drain the pineapple well, reserving the juice. Place the juice in a small pot, and bring to a boil.

2. Place the gelatin mix in a medium-sized heatproof bowl and add the boiling juice. Stir the mixture with a wire whisk for at least 1 minute, until the gelatin is completely dissolved. Set aside for 10 minutes to cool slightly.

3. Stir in the cottage cheese, pineapple, oranges, and pecans. Refrigerate for 15 minutes, or until the mixture is the consistency of pudding. Stir well and then fold in the whipped topping. Pour the mixture into a 2-quart glass dish and chill for several hours before serving.

Nutritional Facts (per serving)

CALORIES: 132 CARBOHYDRATES: 13 g CHOLESTEROL: 3 mg FAT: 5 g SAT. FAT: 0.5 g FIBER: 1.4 g PROTEIN: 7 g SODIUM: 175 mg CALCIUM: 30 mg

Diabetic exchanges: ½ very lean meat, 1 fruit, ½ fat

■ ■ ■

12. SIMPLY GREAT SIDE DISHES

Side dishes present a terrific opportunity to add health-promoting vegetables and whole grains to meals. The problem is convenience often drives our side dish choices, which is why prepackaged potato and rice mixes are featured fare on many dinner tables while fresh vegetables and whole grains are often lacking.

Busy cooks will be happy to know that the less you do to vegetables in the way of cooking, the better off your side dishes will be nutritionally. Simple cooking methods like steaming, roasting, sautéing, and stir-frying are superior techniques for preserving nutrients.

It's also a simple matter to base your side dishes on wholesome whole grains like brown rice, bulgur wheat, barley, and whole-wheat couscous. When combined with plenty of vegetables, some garlic and herbs, and a little olive oil, you can create savory side dishes that are special enough for any occasion.

Be sure to consider your personal nutrition needs when selecting side dishes. For instance, if you are having a starchy entrée like Meat & Potato Pie (p. 210), pair it with a fresh garden salad and a serving of low-carb vegetables such as sautéed zucchini, green beans, or asparagus. Add another starchy food like a piece of hearty whole-grain bread only if you need the extra carbohydrates and calories.

Sicilian-style Asparagus

YIELD: 5 SERVINGS

1 ¼ pounds fresh asparagus spears
Olive oil cooking spray
¼ cup oatmeal or sourdough breadcrumbs*
¼ cup grated Parmesan cheese
2 teaspoons extra virgin olive oil

1. Preheat oven to 450°.

2. Rinse the asparagus with cool water. Shake the excess water off the asparagus and snap off the tough stem ends.

3. Coat an 11 × 13-inch roasting pan or the bottom of a large broiler pan with the cooking spray and spread the asparagus spears in an even layer over the bottom of the pan. Spray the top of the asparagus lightly with the cooking spray and bake uncovered for 8 minutes or until the asparagus is almost tender.

4. While the asparagus is baking, place the breadcrumbs, Parmesan cheese, and olive oil in a small bowl and toss to mix well. Sprinkle the crumb mixture over the asparagus spears and bake for an additional 3 to 4 minutes, until the asparagus is tender and the topping is lightly browned. Serve hot.

Nutritional Facts (per serving)

CALORIES: 67 CARBOHYDRATES: 6 g CHOLESTEROL: 4 mg FAT: 3.6 g SAT. FAT: 1.2 g FIBER: 2 g PROTEIN: 5 g SODIUM: 112 mg CALCIUM: 91 mg

Diabetic exchanges: 1 vegetable, ½ fat

*To make the breadcrumbs, tear about ½ slice of stale firm oatmeal or sourdough bread into small pieces and place in the bowl of a food processor. Process the bread, pulsing the machine for several seconds at a time, until it is ground into crumbs.

■ ■ ■

Broiled Asparagus

YIELD: 4 SERVINGS

1 pound fresh asparagus spears
Olive oil cooking spray or 2 to 3 teaspoons
    extra virgin olive oil
⅛ teaspoon salt
⅛ teaspoon dried thyme or fines herbes

1. Rinse the asparagus with cool water and shake off the excess water. Snap off the tough stem ends.

2. Coat a large baking sheet with nonstick cooking spray and spread the asparagus spears in an even layer over the sheet.

3. Spray the asparagus spears lightly with the cooking spray or drizzle with the olive oil. Sprinkle with the salt, pepper, and herbs and shake the pan to distribute the seasonings. Broil for about 8 minutes, shaking the pan every 3 minutes, or until the spears are tender and lightly browned. Serve hot, topping each serving with a sprinkling of Parmesan cheese or a squeeze of lemon juice if desired.

Nutritional Facts (per serving)

CALORIES: 32 CARBOHYDRATES: 5 g CHOLESTEROL: 0 mg
FAT: 0.2 g SAT. FAT: 0 g FIBER: 2.4 g PROTEIN: 2 g
SODIUM: 91 mg CALCIUM: 25 mg

Diabetic exchanges: 1 vegetable

■ ■ ■

Easy Oven-baked Vegetables

YIELD: 5 SERVINGS

1 pound frozen broccoli, cauliflower, and carrot
  medley, or your favorite combination
¼ teaspoon salt
1 teaspoon dried parsley or salt-free herb blend
1 tablespoon extra virgin olive oil

1. Preheat oven to 400°.
2. Coat a 9 × 13-inch pan with nonstick cooking spray and place the frozen vegetables in the dish. Sprinkle with the salt and herbs and toss to mix well. Drizzle with the olive oil and toss to mix.
3. Cover the pan with aluminum foil and bake for about 20 to 25 minutes, or until steaming hot and tender. Serve hot.

Nutritional Facts (per ⅔-cup serving)

CALORIES: 50 CARBOHYDRATES: 5 g CHOLESTEROL: 0 mg
FAT: 2.9 g SAT. FAT: 0.4 g FIBER: 2.6 g PROTEIN: 2 g
SODIUM: 91 mg CALCIUM: 33 mg

Diabetic exchanges: 1 vegetable, ½ fat

■ ■ ■

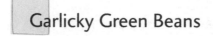

Garlicky Green Beans

YIELD: 5 SERVINGS

1 pound frozen French-cut green beans
2 tablespoons water
¼ teaspoon dried thyme
¼ teaspoon salt
1 tablespoon extra virgin olive oil
1½ teaspoons crushed garlic

1. Place the frozen green beans, water, thyme, and salt in a large nonstick skillet. Cover and cook over medium-high heat, stirring occasionally, for about 7 minutes, until the green beans are completely thawed. Reduce the heat to medium and cook for several minutes more, just until tender. (Add a little more water during cooking if needed, but only enough to prevent scorching.) Drain off any excess liquid.
2. Push the beans to one side of the skillet and add the olive oil and garlic to the empty side of the skillet. Increase the heat to medium-high and cook for about 10 seconds, until the garlic smells fragrant and is just beginning to turn color. Toss the beans with the garlic mixture and serve hot.

Nutritional Facts (per ⅔-cup serving)

CALORIES: 54 CARBOHYDRATES: 7 g CHOLESTEROL: 0 mg
FAT: 2.8 g SAT. FAT: 0.4 g FIBER: 2.5 g PROTEIN: 1.6 g
SODIUM: 119 mg CALCIUM: 38 mg

Diabetic exchanges: 1½ vegetable, ½ fat

▪ ▪ ▪

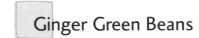Green Beans with Almonds

YIELD: 5 SERVINGS

1 pound frozen French-cut green beans
1 tablespoon margarine or butter
3 tablespoons sliced almonds
½ teaspoon dried dill
¼ teaspoon salt

1. Cook the green beans according to package directions, just until tender. Drain off the excess liquid.

2. Place the margarine or butter in a large nonstick skillet and melt over medium heat. Add the almonds and sauté for about 1 minute, or just until they begin to turn color (be careful not to burn them). Add the green beans, dill, and salt to the almonds and toss to mix. Serve hot.

Nutritional Facts (per ⅔-cup serving)

CALORIES: 68 CARBOHYDRATES: 7 g CHOLESTEROL: 0 mg
FAT: 3.9 g SAT. FAT: 0.7 g FIBER: 2.9 g PROTEIN: 2.5 g
SODIUM: 138 mg CALCIUM: 46 mg

Diabetic exchanges: 1 vegetable, 1 fat

▪ ▪ ▪

Ginger Green Beans

YIELD: 5 SERVINGS

1 tablespoon canola oil
4 cups 1½-inch pieces fresh green beans
2 tablespoons water
1 medium-large yellow onion, thinly sliced
½ teaspoon ground ginger
1 teaspoon crushed garlic
2 tablespoons light teriyaki sauce

1. Place the oil in a large nonstick skillet. Add the green beans and water and place over medium heat. Cover and cook for 4 minutes, shaking the pan occasionally. Add the onions, cover, and cook for an additional 4 minutes, until the green beans are tender and the onions are lightly browned. Add a little more water during cooking if needed, but only enough to prevent scorching.

2. Add the ginger, garlic, and teriyaki sauce. Cover and cook over low heat for a minute or two to blend the flavors. If necessary, cook uncovered for a minute or two to evaporate any excess liquid. Serve hot.

Nutritional Facts (per ⅔-cup serving)

CALORIES: 62 CARBOHYDRATES: 8 g CHOLESTEROL: 0 mg
FAT: 2.8 g SAT. FAT: 0.2 g FIBER: 3 g PROTEIN: 1.6 g
SODIUM: 129 mg CALCIUM: 42 mg

Diabetic exchanges: 1½ vegetable, ½ fat

▪ ▪ ▪

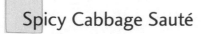 Spicy Cabbage Sauté

YIELD: 6 SERVINGS

1 tablespoon extra virgin olive oil

1 medium yellow onion, thinly sliced

2 medium carrots, shredded with a potato
   peeler

½ medium head cabbage, cut into 2-inch
   wedges and sliced ½-inch thick

1 teaspoon curry powder or curry paste

¼ teaspoon salt

¼ cup chicken or vegetable broth

1. Coat a large nonstick skillet with the olive oil and add the onion and carrots. Place the skillet over medium heat, cover, and cook for several minutes, until the vegetables start to soften. (Add a little water if the skillet becomes too dry.)

2. Add the remaining ingredients to the skillet. Cover and cook, stirring occasionally, for about 5 minutes, until the cabbage is wilted and tender. Add a little more broth during cooking if necessary, but only enough to prevent scorching. Serve hot.

———————

Nutritional Facts (per ⅔-cup serving)
CALORIES: 54 CARBOHYDRATES: 7 g CHOLESTEROL: 0 mg
FAT: 2.5 g SAT. FAT: 0.3 g FIBER: 2.9 g PROTEIN: 1.2 g
SODIUM: 146 mg CALCIUM: 54 mg
   Diabetic exchanges: 1½ vegetable, ½ fat

■ ■ ■

Honey-glazed Carrots

YIELD: 6 SERVINGS

1 pound baby carrots

½ cup water

⅛ teaspoon salt

1 tablespoon margarine or butter

2 tablespoons honey

1. Place the carrots, water, and salt in a large, nonstick skillet and bring to a boil over medium-high heat. Reduce the heat to medium, cover, and cook for about 7 minutes, just until tender. Add a little more water during cooking if the skillet becomes too dry, but only enough to prevent scorching.

2. Add the margarine or butter and the honey and raise the heat to medium-high. Cook, stirring frequently, for another minute or two, until most of the liquid evaporates and the carrots are coated with the glaze. Serve hot.

———————

Nutritional Facts (per ½-cup serving)
CALORIES: 63 CARBOHYDRATES: 12 g CHOLESTEROL: 0
mg FAT: 1.9 g SAT. FAT: 0.5 g FIBER: 2 g PROTEIN: 0.7 g
SODIUM: 90 mg CALCIUM: 18 mg
   Diabetic exchanges: 1 vegetable, ⅓ other carbohydrate, ½ fat

■ ■ ■

Cauliflower with Mushrooms & Onions

YIELD: 5 SERVINGS

5 cups fresh cauliflower florets (about 1 medium head)
1 medium yellow onion, sliced ½-inch thick and separated into rings
2 cups sliced fresh mushrooms
¼ teaspoon salt
⅛ teaspoon ground black pepper
1 tablespoon extra virgin olive oil

1. Preheat oven to 425°.
2. Coat an 11 × 13-inch roasting pan or the bottom of a large broiler pan with nonstick cooking spray and place the cauliflower, onion rings, and mushrooms in the pan. Sprinkle the vegetables with the salt and pepper and drizzle with the olive oil. Toss to mix well.
3. Cover the pan with aluminum foil and bake for 10 minutes. Remove the foil and bake for an additional 15 to 20 minutes, stirring every 5 minutes, or until the vegetables are tender and lightly browned. Serve hot.

Nutritional Facts (per ¾-cup serving)
CALORIES: 64 CARBOHYDRATES: 8 g CHOLESTEROL: 0 mg
FAT: 3 g SAT. FAT: 0.4 g FIBER: 3.2 g PROTEIN: 3 g
SODIUM: 148 mg CALCIUM: 28 mg
Diabetic exchanges: 1½ vegetable, ½ fat

■ ■ ■

Herb-roasted Corn

YIELD: 6 SERVINGS

1½ teaspoons dried parsley, finely crumbled
¼ teaspoon garlic powder
¼ teaspoon salt
¼ teaspoon ground black pepper
6 medium-sized ears fresh corn, shucked
Olive oil- or butter-flavored cooking spray

1. Preheat oven to 450°.
2. Combine the parsley, garlic powder, salt, and pepper in a small bowl and stir to mix well. Set aside.
3. Arrange the ears of corn on a large nonstick baking sheet. Spray all sides of the ears with the cooking spray and sprinkle each ear with some of the spice mixture.
4. Bake for 15 minutes, turn the ears over, and bake for an additional 10 to 15 minutes, until the kernels are tender and lightly browned. Serve hot.

Nutritional Facts (per serving)
CALORIES: 92 CARBOHYDRATES: 19 g CHOLESTEROL: 0 mg
FAT: 2 g SAT. FAT: 0.2 g FIBER: 2.2 g PROTEIN: 2.6 g
SODIUM: 110 mg CALCIUM: 7 mg
Diabetic exchanges: 1 starch

■ ■ ■

Stuffed Portabella Mushrooms

YIELD: 4 SERVINGS

4 medium-large portabella mushrooms
½ cup finely chopped yellow onion
⅛ teaspoon dried thyme
3 cups chopped fresh spinach
½ teaspoon crushed garlic
2 tablespoons chopped sun-dried tomatoes
    packed in olive oil, drained
½ cup cooked whole-wheat couscous or
    brown rice
¼ cup grated Parmesan cheese
Olive oil nonstick cooking spray

1. Preheat oven to 450°.
2. Trim the stems from the mushrooms and use a spoon to scrape out the gills, creating a shallow depression in each mushroom. Set aside.
3. Coat a large nonstick skillet with nonstick cooking spray and add the onions and thyme. Place the skillet over medium heat, cover, and cook for several minutes, until the onions are tender. (Add a little water during cooking if the skillet becomes too dry.) Add the spinach and garlic and sauté for a minute or two, until the spinach is wilted. Remove the skillet from the heat and stir in the sun-dried tomatoes, couscous, and Parmesan cheese.
4. Place a quarter of the spinach mixture

in the depression in each mushroom cap, mounding the top slightly. Spray the tops lightly with the cooking spray. Place the stuffed mushrooms on a large baking sheet and bake uncovered at 450 degrees for 15 minutes, until the mushrooms are tender and the topping is lightly browned. Serve hot.

Nutritional Facts (per serving)
CALORIES: 87 CARBOHYDRATES: 10 g CHOLESTEROL: 5 mg FAT: 2.5 g SAT. FAT: 1.3 g FIBER: 2 g PROTEIN: 4.9 g SODIUM: 146 mg CALCIUM: 115 mg
    Diabetic exchanges: 2 vegetable, ½ fat

■ ■ ■

Summer Garden Pilaf

For variety, substitute bulgur wheat or whole-wheat couscous for the rice.

YIELD: 7 SERVINGS

1 tablespoon extra virgin olive oil or canola oil
1 cup plus 2 tablespoons (⅓-inch dice) zucchini
1 cup fresh or frozen whole kernel corn
½ cup chopped red bell pepper
½ cup chopped onion
½ teaspoon dried oregano
3 cups cooked brown rice
Scant ½ teaspoon salt

1. Place the oil in a large deep nonstick skillet and preheat over medium-high heat. Add the zucchini, corn, red bell pepper, onion,

and oregano. Cook, stirring frequently, for 3 to 4 minutes, just until the vegetables are crisp-tender. Periodically place a lid over the skillet if it becomes too dry. (The steam released from the cooking vegetables will moisten the skillet.)

2. Add the rice and salt to the skillet mixture and reduce the heat to medium. Cook, stirring frequently, for a couple of minutes, until the mixture is heated through. Add a tablespoon or two of water if the mixture seems too dry. Serve hot.

Nutritional Facts (per ¾-cup serving)
CALORIES: 140 CARBOHYDRATES: 26 g
CHOLESTEROL: 0 mg FAT: 2.9 g SAT. FAT: 0.4 g
FIBER: 2.7 g PROTEIN: 3.3 g SODIUM: 138 mg
CALCIUM: 16 mg
   Diabetic exchanges: 1¼ starch, 1 vegetable, ½ fat

■ ■ ■

Colorful Rice Pilaf

YIELD: 6 SERVINGS

2 tablespoons reduced-fat margarine or
   light butter
½ cup finely chopped celery
½ cup thinly sliced scallions
½ cup finely chopped carrot
3 cups cooked brown rice
¼ teaspoon salt
1 tablespoon finely chopped fresh parsley or
   1 teaspoon dried

1. Place the margarine or butter in a large nonstick skillet and preheat over medium heat. Add the celery, scallions, and carrots. Cover and cook, stirring occasionally, for several minutes, until the vegetables are tender.

2. Add the rice, salt, and parsley to the skillet mixture and cook, stirring frequently, for a couple of minutes, until the mixture is heated through. Add a tablespoon or two of water if the mixture seems too dry. Serve hot.

Nutritional Facts (per ⅔-cup serving)
CALORIES: 132 CARBOHYDRATES: 24 g
CHOLESTEROL: 0 mg FAT: 2.6 g SAT. FAT: 0.7 g
FIBER: 2.6 g PROTEIN: 2.7 g SODIUM: 149 mg
CALCIUM: 17 mg
   Diabetic exchanges: 1¼ starch, ½ vegetable, ½ fat

■ ■ ■

Dilled New Potatoes & Peas

YIELD: 5 SERVINGS

3 cups 1-inch chunks new potatoes (about
   1 pound)
1⅛ cups frozen green peas
1 tablespoon extra virgin olive oil
1 to 1½ tablespoons finely chopped fresh dill or
   1 to 1½ teaspoons dried
¼ teaspoon salt

1. Place the potatoes in a 4-quart pot, cover with water, and bring to a boil over high heat. Reduce the heat to medium and cook

for about 10 minutes, until the potatoes are tender. Add the peas and cook for another minute, until the peas are heated through. Drain the potatoes and peas and return them to the pot.

2. Add the olive oil, dill, and salt to the potatoes and peas and toss to mix well. Serve hot.

Nutritional Facts (per ¾-cup serving)
CALORIES: 129 CARBOHYDRATES: 23 g CHOLESTEROL: 0 mg FAT: 2.9 g SAT. FAT: 0.4 g FIBER: 3.3 g PROTEIN: 3.4 g SODIUM: 159 mg CALCIUM: 18 mg
Diabetic exchanges: 1½ starch, ½ fat

■ ■ ■

Roasted Root Vegetables

YIELD: 7 SERVINGS

1 pound new potatoes, cut into ¾-inch chunks
1 pound baby carrots
2 medium-large yellow onions, cut into
   1-inch wedges
1½ tablespoons extra virgin olive oil
1 teaspoon fines herbes or ¼ teaspoon each
   thyme, sage, oregano, and rosemary
Scant ½ teaspoon salt
¼ teaspoon coarsely ground black pepper

1. Preheat oven to 450°.
2. Place all of the ingredients in a large bowl and toss to mix well.
3. Coat an 11 × 13-inch nonstick roast-

ing pan or the bottom of a large broiler pan with nonstick cooking spray and spread the vegetable mixture over the bottom of the pan.

4. Bake for 10 minutes, stir the vegetables, and cook for an additional 20 minutes, stirring every 5 minutes, until the vegetables are tender and nicely browned. Serve hot.

Nutritional Facts (per 1-cup serving)
CALORIES: 119 CARBOHYDRATES: 21 g CHOLESTEROL: 0 mg FAT: 3.3 g SAT. FAT: 0.5 g FIBER: 3 g PROTEIN: 2.1 g SODIUM: 160 mg CALCIUM: 26 mg
Diabetic exchanges: 1 starch, 1 vegetable, ½ fat

■ ■ ■

Garlic Smashed New Potatoes

YIELD: 6 SERVINGS

1½ pounds unpeeled red-skinned new potatoes,
   scrubbed and cut into 1-inch chunks
4 to 6 cloves peeled garlic
½ cup light sour cream
¼ teaspoon salt

1. Place the potatoes and garlic in a large pot and cover with water. Bring to a boil, then reduce the heat to medium, cover, and cook for about 15 minutes, until tender. Drain the potatoes, reserving ¼ cup of the cooking liquid.

2. Pick out the garlic cloves from the potatoes, place in a medium bowl, and mash

with a fork. Add the sour cream and reserved cooking liquid to the garlic and stir until smooth. Add the sour cream mixture and the salt to the potatoes and stir to mix. Mash the potatoes with a potato masher just enough to make them creamy but still with good sized chunks of potatoes. Serve hot.

Nutritional Facts (per ⅔-cup serving)
CALORIES: 126 CARBOHYDRATES: 26 g CHOLESTEROL: 0 mg FAT: 1.2 g SAT. FAT: 0.7 g FIBER: 2.3 g PROTEIN: 3 g SODIUM: 119 mg CALCIUM: 17 mg
Diabetic exchanges: 1½ starch

▪ ▪ ▪

Simply Baked Spaghetti Squash

YIELD: 8 SERVINGS

2¼ to 2½-pound spaghetti squash
2 tablespoons margarine or butter
1 ½ tablespoons honey

1. Preheat oven to 375°.
2. Rinse the squash, cut it in half lengthwise and scoop out the seeds. Coat a large baking sheet with cooking spray and lay the squash halves, cut side down, on the sheet. Bake for about 45 minutes, until the squash can be easily pierced with a fork.
3. Place the margarine or butter and honey in a microwave safe dish, cover loosely, and mi-

crowave at high power for about 30 seconds, until the margarine or butter is melted.
4. Cut each squash half into quarters and use a fork to fluff the center of each piece of squash slightly. Stir the honey mixture and drizzle about 1¼ teaspoons of the mixture over each piece of squash. Serve hot.

Nutritional Facts (per serving)
CALORIES: 62 CARBOHYDRATES: 9 g CHOLESTEROL: 0 mg FAT: 2.9 g SAT. FAT: 0.5 g FIBER: 1.4 g PROTEIN: 0.7 g SODIUM: 55 mg CALCIUM: 20 mg
Diabetic exchanges: 1½ vegetable, ½ fat

▪ ▪ ▪

Spinach & Onion Sauté

YIELD: 4 SERVINGS

2 tablespoons reduced-fat margarine or light butter
1 medium yellow onion, very thinly sliced
¼ teaspoon dried thyme
10-ounce package prewashed baby spinach (about 10 cups)

1. Place the margarine or butter in a large, deep, nonstick skillet. Add the onion and thyme and place over medium heat. Cover and cook for several minutes, until the onions are soft.
2. Add the spinach, and toss gently over medium-high heat for a couple of minutes, just until the spinach is wilted. Serve hot.

Nutritional Facts (per ⅔-cup serving)
CALORIES: 48 CARBOHYDRATES: 5 g CHOLESTEROL: 0 mg
FAT: 2.8 g SAT. FAT: 0.8 g FIBER: 2.3 g PROTEIN: 2.3 g
SODIUM: 106 mg CALCIUM: 75 mg
Diabetic exchanges: 1 vegetable, ½ fat

■ ■ ■

Summer Squash with Onions & Herbs

YIELD: 5 SERVINGS

1 tablespoon extra virgin olive oil or canola oil
1 medium yellow onion, sliced and separated
 into rings
5 cups sliced yellow or zucchini squash
1 teaspoon dried parsley
1 teaspoon dried dill
¼ teaspoon salt

1. Coat a large nonstick skillet with the oil and place over medium heat.

2. Add the remaining ingredients, cover, and cook, stirring occasionally for about 5 minutes, until the squash and onions are just tender. Serve hot.

Nutritional Facts (per ⅔-cup serving)
CALORIES: 56 CARBOHYDRATES: 7 g CHOLESTEROL: 0 mg
FAT: 3 g SAT. FAT: 0.4 g FIBER: 2.7 g PROTEIN: 1.9 g
SODIUM: 119 mg CALCIUM: 32 mg
Diabetic exchanges: 1½ vegetable, ½ fat

■ ■ ■

Roasted Zucchini, Mushrooms, & Onions

YIELD: 4 SERVINGS

3 medium zucchini, halved lengthwise and sliced
 ¼-inch thick (about 1 pound)
1½ cups sliced mushroom
1 medium-large yellow onion, sliced and
 separated into rings
2 to 3 teaspoons extra virgin olive oil
¼ teaspoon salt
½ teaspoon dried Italian seasoning

1. Preheat oven to 450°.

2. Place all of the ingredients in a large bowl and toss to mix well.

3. Coat an 11 × 13-inch roasting pan or the bottom of a broiler pan with nonstick cooking spray and spread vegetable mixture over the bottom of the pan.

4. Bake for 15 minutes. Stir the vegetables and cook for another 5 to 10 minutes, until they are tender and nicely browned. Serve hot.

Nutritional Facts (per ¾-cup serving)
CALORIES: 53 CARBOHYDRATES: 7 g CHOLESTEROL: 0 mg
FAT: 2.5 g SAT. FAT: 0.4 g FIBER: 2.3 g PROTEIN: 2.4 g
SODIUM: 150 mg CALCIUM: 24 mg
Diabetic exchanges: 1 vegetable, ½ fat

■ ■ ■

13. Smart Sandwiches

Mention lunch and most people immediately think of the sandwich. Versatile, portable, and fast and easy to make and eat, sandwiches are hard to beat for folks who are on the run. But how do sandwiches stack up nutritionally? Made right, this grab-and-go meal can be just what the doctor ordered. Sandwiches made with whole-grain bread, lean protein fillings, light spreads, and plenty of vegetable toppings can make for a light and healthy meal. Realize, though, that what you have *with* your sandwich can make or break your meal. Keep your carbohydrate load down by choosing a garden salad, a cup of soup, or fresh fruit instead of starchy accompaniments like chips, fries, and pretzels.

This chapter offers a selection of hearty and creative sandwiches that are a snap to make. Whether you are looking for a veggie-stuffed pita, a creative wrap, or some down-home sloppy joes, you are sure to find a sandwich that meets your need deliciously.

Greek Garden Sandwiches

YIELD: 4 SANDWICHES

10-ounce package frozen chopped spinach,
   thawed and squeezed dry
¼ cup coarsely chopped black olives
¼ cup nonfat or light mayonnaise
3 tablespoons crumbled reduced-fat feta cheese
   with sun-dried tomatoes and herbs
8 slices firm multigrain, pumpernickel, or dark
   rye bread or 4 multigrain burger buns
12 thin slices plum tomato
¾ cup alfalfa or spicy sprouts
4 ounces thinly sliced reduced-fat provolone or
   Swiss cheese
2 tablespoons Dijon mustard

1. Put the spinach in a large nonstick skillet and place over medium heat. Cook, stirring frequently, until the spinach is heated through and any excess liquid has evaporated. Remove the skillet from the heat and stir in first the olives and mayonnaise, and then the feta cheese.

2. To assemble the sandwiches, place a quarter of the spinach mixture on each of four bread slices. Top the spinach on each bread slice with a quarter of the tomatoes, sprouts, and cheese. Spread the remaining 4 bread slices with some of the mustard and place on the sandwiches.

3. Place each sandwich on a microwave-safe plate and cover with a paper towel. Microwave at high power for about 30 seconds, just until the cheese is melted. Serve hot.

Nutritional Facts (per serving)
CALORIES: 276 CARBOHYDRATES: 32 g
CHOLESTEROL: 17 mg FAT: 8.6 g SAT. FAT: 3.1 g
FIBER: 6.3 g PROTEIN: 19 g SODIUM: 905 mg
CALCIUM: 415 mg
   Diabetic exchanges: 2 starch, 1 lean meat,
1 vegetable, 1 fat

■ ■ ■

Chicken Gyros

YIELD: 4 SERVINGS

SAUCE
1 cup plain low-fat yogurt or light sour cream
¾ cup peeled, seeded, finely chopped cucumber
½ teaspoon dried dill

1 pound boneless skinless chicken breast, cut
   into thin strips
1 teaspoon lemon pepper
½ teaspoon dried oregano
¼ teaspoon garlic powder
1 tablespoon extra virgin olive oil
4 whole-wheat or oat-bran pita pockets (6-inch
   rounds), cut in half
8 leaves romaine lettuce
2 medium-small plum tomatoes, thinly sliced
4 slices red onion, separated into rings

1. Combine all of the sauce ingredients and stir to mix well. Cover and refrigerate until ready to use.

2. Combine the chicken, lemon pepper, oregano, and garlic powder in a medium bowl and toss to mix well. Coat a large nonstick skillet with the olive oil and preheat over medium-high heat. Add the chicken and stir-fry for several minutes, until nicely browned and no longer pink inside. Remove the skillet from the heat and set aside.

3. To heat the pita pockets, place them on a microwave-safe plate. Cover with a damp paper towel and microwave on high power for about 45 seconds. If heating only one pita at a time, microwave for only 15 seconds.

4. To assemble the sandwiches, line each pita half with a lettuce leaf, add some of the chicken, tomatoes, onion slices, and sauce. Serve hot.

Nutritional Facts (per serving)

CALORIES: 346 CARBOHYDRATES: 40 g
CHOLESTEROL: 69 mg FAT: 6.4 g SAT. FAT: 1.5 g
FIBER: 5.4 g PROTEIN: 36 g SODIUM: 544 mg
CALCIUM: 182 mg

Diabetic exchanges: 2 starch, 3 very lean meat, 1 vegetable, ¼ low-fat milk, 1 fat

▪ ▪ ▪

Unfried Fish Sandwiches

YIELD: 4 SERVINGS

SAUCE

¼ cup nonfat or reduced-fat mayonnaise
2 to 3 teaspoons dill or sweet pickle relish
2 teaspoons finely chopped onion
¼ teaspoon dry mustard

FISH

1 pound cod, grouper, orange roughy, or other white fish fillets, cut into 4 equal pieces
¼ cup plus 2 tablespoons fat-free egg substitute
½ cup Special-K cereal crumbs
½ to 1 teaspoon lemon pepper, Cajun seasoning, or Old Bay seafood seasoning
nonstick cooking spray

4 light whole-wheat or multigrain buns
4 slices tomato
4 lettuce leaves

1. Preheat oven to 450°.

2. To make the sauce, combine all of the sauce ingredients in a small bowl and stir to mix well. Cover the dish and refrigerate until ready to serve.

3. Rinse the fish pieces with cool water and pat dry with paper towels. Set aside.

4. Place the egg substitute in a shallow bowl. Place the crumbs and lemon pepper or

seasoning in another shallow bowl and stir to mix well.

5. Coat a large baking sheet with nonstick cooking spray. Dip the fish pieces first in the egg substitute and then in the crumb mixture, turning to coat both sides well.

6. Lay the fish pieces on the coated sheet. Spray the tops lightly with the cooking spray. Bake for about 15 minutes, until the outside is crisp and golden and the fish flakes easily with a fork.

7. To serve, place one fish fillet in each bun. Top with some of the sauce, lettuce, and tomato and serve immediately.

Nutritional Facts (per serving)

CALORIES: 237 CARBOHYDRATES: 31 g
CHOLESTEROL: 48 mg FAT: 3.3 g SAT. FAT: 0.2 g
FIBER: 5.7 g PROTEIN: 29 g SODIUM: 543 mg
CALCIUM: 70 mg

Diabetic exchanges: 2 starch, 3 very lean meat, ½ vegetable

■ ■ ■

Mediterranean Tuna Melts

YIELD: 4 SERVINGS

12-ounce can water-packed chunk-light or
 albacore tuna, drained
1 cup canned artichoke hearts, drained and
 chopped
⅓ cup chopped red onion
½ cup nonfat or light mayonnaise
¼ teaspoon Italian seasoning

¼ teaspoon ground black pepper
4 whole-wheat or oat-bran English muffins, split
 and toasted
⅓ cup grated Parmesan cheese

1. Combine the tuna, artichoke hearts, onion, mayonnaise, Italian seasoning, and pepper in a medium-sized bowl and stir to mix well. Add a little more mayonnaise if the mixture seems too dry.

2. Arrange the English muffins on a baking sheet, split side up. Spread about ¼ cup of the tuna mixture over each piece and place under a preheated broiler for 2 to 3 minutes, until the tuna mixture is heated through. Top each muffin half with 2 teaspoons of the cheese and broil for another minute or two, until the tops are lightly browned. Serve hot.

Nutritional Facts (per serving)

CALORIES: 310 CARBOHYDRATES: 36 g
CHOLESTEROL: 36 mg FAT: 4.6 g SAT. FAT: 2 g
FIBER: 7.1 g PROTEIN: 31 g SODIUM: 991 mg
CALCIUM: 316 mg

Diabetic exchanges: 2 starch, 3 lean meat, ½ vegetable

■ ■ ■

Colossal Club Wraps

YIELD: 4 SERVINGS

4 whole-wheat flour tortillas (8- to 9-inch rounds)
¼ cup nonfat or light mayonnaise
8 ounces thinly sliced roasted turkey breast

4 ounces thinly sliced nonfat or reduced-fat
   cheddar or Swiss cheese

4 slices crisp-cooked turkey bacon

8 thin slices tomato

4 leaves romaine lettuce

1. Warm the tortillas according to the package directions. Lay the tortillas on a flat surface and spread each one with a tablespoon of the mayonnaise, extending the mayonnaise to within ½-inch of the edges.

2. Top the *bottom half only* of each tortilla with a quarter of the turkey, a quarter of the cheese, 1 bacon slice, 2 tomato slices, and a lettuce leaf, leaving a 1½-inch margin on the right and left sides.

3. Fold the right and left margins in, then roll each tortilla up from the bottom to enclose the filling. Cut each wrap in half and serve immediately.

Nutritional Facts (per serving)

CALORIES: 295 CARBOHYDRATES: 31 g
CHOLESTEROL: 60 mg FAT: 3.8 g SAT. FAT: 0.9 g
FIBER: 2.4 g PROTEIN: 32 g SODIUM: 950 mg CALCIUM: 268 mg

   Diabetic exchanges: 2 starch, 3½ very lean meat

▪ ▪ ▪

Mediterranean Turkey Wraps

YIELD: 4 SERVINGS

4 whole-wheat flour tortillas (8- to 9-inch rounds)

¼ cup nonfat or light mayonnaise

8 ounces thinly sliced roasted turkey breast

½ cup diced roasted red bell pepper

½ cup marinated artichoke hearts, drained and
   chopped

¼ cup plus 2 tablespoons crumbled reduced-fat
   feta cheese flavored with herbs and sun-dried
   tomatoes

16 large fresh spinach leaves or 4 leaves romaine
   lettuce

1. Warm the tortillas according to package directions. Lay the tortillas on a flat surface and spread each one with a tablespoon of the mayonnaise, extending the mayonnaise to within ½-inch of the edges.

2. Top the *bottom half only* of each tortilla with a quarter of the turkey, roasted red bell peppers, artichoke hearts, feta cheese, and spinach or romaine, leaving a 1½-inch margin on the right and left sides.

3. Fold the right and left margins in, then roll each tortilla up from the bottom to enclose the filling. Cut each wrap in half and serve immediately.

Nutritional Facts (per serving)
CALORIES: 271 CARBOHYDRATES: 30 g
CHOLESTEROL: 50 mg FAT: 5.8 g SAT. FAT: 1.8 g
FIBER: 3.3 g PROTEIN: 24 g SODIUM: 749 mg
CALCIUM: 66 mg
    Diabetic exchanges: 2 starch, 2½ lean meat,
½ vegetable

■ ■ ■

Turkey & Artichoke Wraps

YIELD: 4 SERVINGS

1 cup finely chopped canned (drained)
    artichoke hearts
2 tablespoons nonfat or light mayonnaise
4 whole-wheat flour tortillas (8- to 9-inch
    rounds)
¼ cup plus 2 tablespoons nonfat or light scallion
    and chive flavored cream cheese
8 ounces thinly sliced roasted turkey breast
8 thin slices plum tomato or red bell pepper
    rings
4 leaves romaine lettuce

    1. Combine the artichoke hearts and mayonnaise in a small bowl and stir to mix well. Set aside.

    2. Warm the tortillas according to package directions. Lay the tortillas on a flat surface and spread each one with 1½ tablespoons of the cream cheese, extending the cream cheese to within 1 inch of the edges.

    3. Top the *bottom half only* of each tortilla

with a quarter of the turkey, a quarter of the artichoke mixture, 2 tomato slices or red bell pepper rings, and a lettuce leaf, leaving a 1½-inch margin on the right and left sides.

    4. Fold the right and left margins in, then roll each tortilla up from the bottom to enclose the filling. Cut each wrap in half and serve immediately.

Nutritional Facts (per serving)
CALORIES: 282 CARBOHYDRATES: 34 g
CHOLESTEROL: 62 mg FAT: 6 g SAT. FAT: 2.5 g
FIBER: 4.8 g PROTEIN: 24 g SODIUM: 574 mg
CALCIUM: 63 mg
    Diabetic exchanges: 2 starch, 2 lean meat,
½ vegetable

■ ■ ■

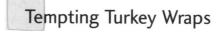

Tempting Turkey Wraps

YIELD: 4 SERVINGS

4 whole-wheat flour tortillas (8- to 9-inch rounds)
¼ cup plus 2 tablespoons light scallion and chive
    or vegetable-flavored cream cheese
8 ounces thinly sliced roasted turkey breast
2 slices red onion, separated into rings
1 small carrot, shredded with a potato peeler
1 cup shredded romaine lettuce

    1. Warm the tortillas according to package directions. Lay the tortillas on a flat surface, and spread *the lower half only* of each tortilla with 1½ tablespoons of the cream cheese.

2. Top the cream cheese on each tortilla with a quarter of the turkey and a quarter of the onion rings, carrots, and lettuce, leaving a 1½-inch margin on the right and left sides.

3. Fold the right and left margins in, then roll each tortilla up from the bottom to enclose the filling. Cut each wrap in half and serve immediately.

Nutritional Facts (per serving)

CALORIES: 269 CARBOHYDRATES: 31 g

CHOLESTEROL: 62 mg FAT: 6 g SAT. FAT: 2.5 g FIBER: 3 g

PROTEIN: 23 g SODIUM: 500 mg CALCIUM: 53 mg

Diabetic exchanges: 2 starch, 2 lean meat, ½ vegetable

▪ ▪ ▪

Chutney Chicken Wraps

YIELD: 4 SERVINGS

2 cups ready-made shredded coleslaw mix

¼ cup nonfat or light mayonnaise

1 tablespoon plus 1 teaspoon mango chutney

4 whole-wheat flour tortillas (8- to 9-inch rounds)

8 ounces thinly sliced roasted chicken or turkey breast

12 fresh spinach leaves or 4 Boston or Bibb lettuce leaves

1. Combine the coleslaw mix, mayonnaise, and chutney and toss to mix well. Set aside.

2. Warm the tortillas according to package directions. Lay the tortillas on a flat surface and layer a quarter of the chicken or turkey over *the lower half only* of each tortilla, leaving a 1½-inch margin on the right and left sides. Top the chicken or turkey on each tortilla with a quarter of the coleslaw mixture followed by the spinach or lettuce.

3. Fold the right and left margins in, then roll each tortilla up from the bottom to enclose the filling. Cut each wrap in half and serve immediately.

Nutritional Facts (per serving)

CALORIES: 262 CARBOHYDRATES: 32 g

CHOLESTEROL: 32 mg FAT: 4.7 g SAT. FAT: 1.1 g

FIBER: 3.1 g PROTEIN: 22 g SODIUM: 535 mg

CALCIUM: 50 mg

Diabetic exchanges: 2 starch, 2 very lean meat, ½ vegetable

▪ ▪ ▪

Hummus-Veggie Wraps

YIELD: 4 SERVINGS

4 whole-wheat flour tortillas (8- to 9-inch rounds)

1 cup Scallion & Olive Hummus (p. 136) or ready-made hummus

1 small carrot, shredded with a potato peeler

2 slices red onion, separated into rings

12 thin slices peeled cucumber

16 young tender spinach leaves or 1 cup alfalfa sprouts

1. Warm the tortillas according to package directions. Lay the tortillas on a flat surface and spread *the lower half only* of each tortilla with ¼ cup of the hummus.

2. Top the hummus on each tortilla with a quarter of the carrots, onion rings, cucumber slices, and spinach or sprouts, leaving a 1½-inch margin on the right and left sides.

3. Fold the right and left margins in, then roll each tortilla up from the bottom to enclose the filling. Cut each wrap in half and serve immediately.

Nutritional Facts (per serving)
CALORIES: 258 CARBOHYDRATES: 38 g
CHOLESTEROL: 0 mg FAT: 8.6 g SAT. FAT: 0.5 g
FIBER: 6.7 g PROTEIN: 10 g SODIUM: 625 mg
CALCIUM: 56 mg
  Diabetic exchanges: 2½ starch, 1 very lean meat, ½ vegetable, 1 fat

■ ■ ■

Teriyaki Turkey Burgers

YIELD: 6 SERVINGS

BURGER MIXTURE
1¼ cups sliced fresh mushrooms
½ cup sliced scallions
½ cup chopped red bell pepper
1¼ pounds 95% lean ground turkey
3 tablespoons light (reduced-sodium) teriyaki sauce
¼ teaspoon ground black pepper

6 canned pineapple rings (optional)
¼ cup plus 2 tablespoons nonfat or light mayonnaise
1 tablespoon Chinese or honey mustard
6 light wheat or multigrain burger buns
6 slices red onion
6 lettuce leaves

1. Place the mushrooms, scallions, and red bell pepper in the bowl of a food processor and process until the vegetables are finely chopped. Place the vegetables, ground turkey, teriyaki sauce, and black pepper in a medium bowl and mix thoroughly. Shape the mixture into six 4-inch patties.

2. Grill the burgers over medium coals or cook under a broiler for about 6 minutes on each side, until the internal temperature of the patties reaches 165 degrees and the meat is no longer pink inside. (To retain moisture, avoid pressing down on the patties as they cook.) Alternatively, coat a large nonstick skillet or griddle with nonstick cooking spray and cook the burgers over medium heat for about 5 minutes per side. If desired, brush the pineapple slices with a little teriyaki sauce and grill or broil for a minute or two on each side, until lightly browned.

3. To assemble the burgers, place the mayonnaise and mustard in a small bowl and stir to mix well. Spread some of the mayonnaise mixture on each bun. Place each burger in a bun and top with some of the onion, lettuce, and if desired, a pineapple slice. Serve hot.

Nutritional Facts (per serving)
CALORIES: 243 CARBOHYDRATES: 29 g
CHOLESTEROL: 50 mg FAT: 5 g SAT. FAT: 1.7 g
FIBER: 6.6 g PROTEIN: 24 g SODIUM: 594 mg
CALCIUM: 61 mg
      Diabetic exchanges: 1½ starch, 2½ lean meat,
1 vegetable

■ ■ ■

Tex-Mex Turkey Burgers

YIELD: 6 SERVINGS

BURGER MIXTURE
1 cup sliced fresh mushrooms
¾ cup chopped zucchini
½ cup chopped onion
½ cup chopped red bell pepper
**1¼ pounds 95% lean ground turkey or
   ground beef**
1½ tablespoons taco seasoning mix

**¾ cup shredded nonfat or reduced-fat Monterey
   Jack or Mexican-blend cheese**
6 light wheat or multigrain burger buns
**¼ cup plus 2 tablespoons salsa or ketchup
   (or mix half and half)**
6 slices red or sweet white onion
6 slices tomato
6 lettuce leaves

1. Place the mushrooms, zucchini, onion, and red bell pepper in the bowl of a food processor and process until the vegetables are finely chopped. Place the vegetables, ground meat, and taco seasoning mix in a medium-sized bowl and mix thoroughly. Shape the mixture into six 4-inch patties.

2. Grill the burgers over medium coals or cook under a broiler for about 6 minutes on each side, until the internal temperature of the patties reaches 165 degrees (160 degrees for ground beef) and the meat is no longer pink inside. (To retain moisture, avoid pressing down on the patties as they cook.) Alternatively, coat a large nonstick skillet or griddle with cooking spray and cook the burgers over medium heat for about 5 minutes per side. Sprinkle 2 tablespoons of the cheese over each burger, cover the grill, and cook for another minute, just until the cheese is melted.

3. Place each burger in a bun and top with some of the salsa or ketchup, onion, tomato, and lettuce. Serve hot.

Nutritional Facts (per serving)
CALORIES: 288 CARBOHYDRATES: 29 g
CHOLESTEROL: 66 mg FAT: 6.3 g SAT. FAT: 1 g FIBER: 6 g
PROTEIN: 32 g SODIUM: 658 mg CALCIUM: 183 mg
      Diabetic exchanges: 1½ starch, 2½ lean meat,
1 vegetable

■ ■ ■

Slimmed-Down Sloppy Joes

YIELD: 6 SERVINGS

1 pound 95% lean ground beef or turkey

1 medium onion, chopped

1 medium green bell pepper, chopped

1 packet (about 1.3 ounces) Sloppy Joe
   seasoning mix

6 ounces tomato paste

1 ¼ cups water

6 light wheat or multigrain burger buns

1. Place the ground meat in a large non-stick skillet. Cook over medium heat, stirring to crumble until the meat is no longer pink. Drain off and discard any fat. Add the onion and pepper, cover, and cook for about 5 minutes, until the vegetables are tender.

2. Add the Sloppy Joe mix, tomato paste, and water, and bring the mixture to a boil, stirring frequently. Reduce the heat to low, cover, and simmer with the lid ajar, for about 10 minutes, stirring occasionally, until the mixture is thick. Spoon the mixture over the buns and serve hot.

Nutritional Facts (per serving)
CALORIES: 237 CARBOHYDRATES: 32 g CHOLESTEROL: 40 mg FAT: 4.1 g SAT. FAT: 1.4 g FIBER: 6 g PROTEIN: 20 g SODIUM: 689 mg CALCIUM: 40 mg
   Diabetic exchanges: 2 starch, 2 lean meat, 1 vegetable

■ ■ ■

Carolina Barbecue Sandwiches

YIELD: 10 SERVINGS

3-pound well-trimmed bone-in pork sirloin roast

½ teaspoon ground black pepper

1 cup low-sodium chicken broth

½ cup roasted garlic-flavored tomato sauce

3 tablespoons apple cider vinegar

3 tablespoons Worcestershire sauce

3 tablespoons dark brown sugar

1 teaspoon dry mustard

½ teaspoon celery seed

10 light wheat or multigrain burger buns

2 cups ready-made low fat coleslaw (optional)

1. Rinse the roast with cool water and pat dry with paper towels. Sprinkle with the pepper. Coat a 6-quart pot with nonstick cooking spray and preheat over medium-high heat. Add the roast and cook for several minutes, until nicely browned on all sides.

2. Combine the broth, tomato sauce, vinegar, Worcestershire sauce, brown sugar, mustard, and celery seed and stir to mix well. Pour the mixture over the roast and bring to a boil. Reduce the heat to low, cover, and simmer for about 2½ hours, until the roast is very tender and shreds easily with a fork. Remove the roast to a large bowl and set aside.

3. Bring the pan juices to a boil over medium-high heat and cook uncovered for about 10 minutes, until the mixture is reduced to about 1¼ cups in volume. Set aside.

4. Using two forks, tear the meat into shreds. Discard the bones and any visible fat. Return the shredded roast to the pan juices and toss to mix well.

5. To assemble the sandwiches, place about ½ cup of the meat mixture on the bottom half of each bun. If desired, top with 3 to 4 tablespoons of coleslaw. Place the tops on the sandwiches and serve hot.

Nutritional Facts (per serving)
CALORIES: 276 CARBOHYDRATES: 33 g
CHOLESTEROL: 62 mg FAT: 4.2 g SAT. FAT: 0.9 g
FIBER: 6 g PROTEIN: 27 g SODIUM: 621 mg
CALCIUM: 65 mg
   Diabetic exchanges: 2 starch, 2½ lean meat, ½ vegetable

▪ ▪ ▪

14. Main Dish Pastabilities

Pasta can be the perfect solution when you need a meal in a matter of minutes. But in recent years, pasta has been shunned by many dieters due to its high carbohydrate content. Is this really necessary? Not if you plan your pasta meals properly.

The dishes in this chapter have been developed with both taste and nutrition in mind. Pasta is combined with lean meats, seafood, plenty of garden vegetables, and light sauces to create an assortment of satisfying dishes that won't blow your fat, calorie, or carbohydrate budgets. To optimize nutrition, most of these dishes suggest using whole-wheat pasta, which is now widely available in grocery stores.

While the pasta entrées in this chapter are healthful choices, realize that like all starchy foods, pasta is a concentrated source of carbohydrates. So when planning pasta meals, be sure to keep your calorie and carbohydrate goals in mind. For instance, if you are watching your weight and your carbohydrate intake, balance your pasta entrée with lower-carb side dishes like a fresh garden salad and some sautéed broccoli or asparagus. Add some crusty whole-grain bread only if you need the extra carbohydrates and calories.

Penne with Sausage, Peppers, & Onions

YIELD: 5 SERVINGS

8 ounces whole-wheat penne pasta

1 pound turkey Italian sausage, sliced

2 medium yellow onions, cut into ½-inch wedges

1 medium green bell pepper, cut into ½-inch strips

1 medium red bell pepper, cut into ½-inch strips

3 cups marinara sauce

Grated Parmesan cheese (optional)

1. Cook the pasta al dente according to package directions. Drain, return to the pot, and set aside to keep warm.

2. While the pasta is cooking, coat a large nonstick skillet with cooking spray and add the sausage. Cook over medium heat, stirring frequently, until the meat is no longer pink. Drain off and discard any fat. Add the onions and peppers to the sausage, cover, and cook, stirring occasionally for several minutes, or until the vegetables are tender. Add the marinara sauce and cook for another minute or two to heat through.

3. Pour the sauce over the pasta and toss to mix well. Serve hot, topping each serving with some Parmesan if desired.

Nutritional Facts (per 1¾-cup serving)
CALORIES: 389 CARBOHYDRATES: 49 g
CHOLESTEROL: 76 mg FAT: 8.3 g SAT. FAT: 2.6 g
FIBER: 8 g PROTEIN: 25 g SODIUM: 838 mg
CALCIUM: 21 mg
  Diabetic exchanges: 2½ starch, 2 vegetable, 2½ lean meat

■ ■ ■

Penne with Chicken, Artichoke Hearts, & Sun-Dried Tomatoes

YIELD: 5 SERVINGS

8 ounces whole-wheat penne pasta

1 pound boneless skinless chicken breast, cut into thin strips

1 teaspoon dried rosemary

½ teaspoon garlic powder

¼ teaspoon salt

1 tablespoon extra virgin olive oil

2 cups sliced baby portabella or button mushrooms

¼ cup plus 2 tablespoons chopped sun-dried tomatoes (not packed in oil)

¼ cup plus 2 tablespoons chicken broth

1 teaspoon cornstarch

1 cup evaporated skim or low-fat milk

¾ cup chopped canned (drained) artichoke hearts

2 tablespoons grated Parmesan cheese

3 tablespoons sliced scallions or finely chopped fresh parsley

1. Cook the pasta al dente according to package directions. Drain, return to the pot, and set aside to keep warm.

2. Toss the chicken with the rosemary, garlic powder, and salt. Set aside. Coat a large nonstick skillet with the olive oil and preheat over medium-high heat. Add the chicken and cook, stirring frequently, for several minutes, until the meat is nicely browned and no longer pink inside. Add the mushrooms to the skillet, cover, and cook for a couple of minutes, until tender.

3. Add the sun-dried tomatoes and broth to the skillet, reduce the heat to medium, cover, and cook for a couple of minutes, until the broth is absorbed and the tomatoes have plumped. Dissolve the cornstarch into a tablespoon of the evaporated milk then mix with the remaining milk. Pour the mixture into the skillet and cook, stirring frequently, until the mixture boils and thickens slightly.

4. Add the artichoke hearts and pasta to the skillet mixture and toss over low heat to mix well. Remove the skillet from the heat and toss in the Parmesan cheese. Serve hot, topping each serving with some of the scallions or parsley.

Nutritional Facts (per 1¾-cup serving)
CALORIES: 373 CARBOHYDRATES: 46 g
CHOLESTEROL: 56 mg FAT: 5.6 g SAT. FAT: 1.4 g
FIBER: 5.9 g PROTEIN: 33 g SODIUM: 419 mg
CALCIUM: 220 mg
   Diabetic exchanges: 2½ starch, 1½ vegetable, 2½ very lean meat, ½ fat, ½ nonfat milk

Rotini with Savory-Meat Sauce

YIELD: 6 SERVINGS

10 ounces whole-wheat rotini, penne,
   or rigatoni pasta
1 pound 95% lean ground beef
2 cups sliced fresh mushrooms
¾ cup chopped onion
½ cup chopped red or green bell pepper
26-ounce jar marinara sauce

1. Cook the pasta al dente according to package directions. Drain, return to the pot, and set aside to keep warm.

2. While the pasta is cooking, coat a large nonstick skillet with nonstick cooking spray and add the ground beef. Cook over medium heat, stirring frequently, until the meat is no longer pink. Drain off and discard any fat. Add the mushrooms, onions, and peppers to the skillet, cover, and cook, stirring occasionally for several minutes, until the mushrooms are tender. Add the marinara sauce and cook for another minute or two to heat through.

3. To serve, place 1 cup of pasta on each of 6 serving plates and top with about ⅞ cup of the sauce. Serve hot, topping each serving with some grated Parmesan cheese if desired.

Nutritional Facts (per serving)

CALORIES: 325 CARBOHYDRATES: 45 g

CHOLESTEROL: 40 mg FAT: 4.2 g SAT. FAT: 1.5 g

FIBER: 5.5 g PROTEIN: 24 g SODIUM: 449 mg

CALCIUM: 15 mg

Diabetic exchanges: 2½ starch, 1½ vegetable, 2½ lean meat

■ ■ ■

Primavera Pasta

YIELD: 4 SERVINGS

6 ounces whole-wheat thin spaghetti

1½ cups 1-inch pieces fresh asparagus

½ cup frozen green peas

1 tablespoon plus 1 teaspoon extra virgin olive oil

4 ounces thinly sliced lean ham, cut into
    thin strips

1 cup diced zucchini

1 teaspoon dried Italian seasoning

½ teaspoon coarsely ground black pepper

1½ teaspoons crushed garlic

½ cup halved grape tomatoes

½ cup chicken broth

¼ cup dry white wine

¼ cup grated Parmesan cheese

1. Cook the spaghetti al dente according to package directions. Two minutes before the pasta is done, add the asparagus and peas. Drain well and return to the pot.

2. Coat a large nonstick skillet with the olive oil and preheat over medium-high heat.

Add the ham, zucchini, Italian seasoning, and pepper, and sauté for several minutes, until the ham is beginning to brown and the zucchini is crisp-tender. Add the garlic and tomatoes and cook for another minute, until the tomatoes are heated through and just beginning to soften. Transfer the ham and vegetables to the pot containing the spaghetti and set aside.

3. Add the broth and wine to the skillet and bring to a boil. Cook, stirring frequently, for several minutes, until the liquid is reduced by half. Add the pasta, ham, and vegetables back to the skillet and toss over low heat for a minute or two to heat through. Remove the skillet from the heat and toss in the Parmesan cheese. Serve hot.

Nutritional Facts (per 1¾-cup serving)

CALORIES: 307 CARBOHYDRATES: 42 g

CHOLESTEROL: 13 mg FAT: 8.2 g SAT. FAT: 2.2 g

FIBER: 6.6 g PROTEIN: 16 g SODIUM: 489 mg

CALCIUM: 116 mg

Diabetic exchanges: 2½ starch, 1 vegetable, 1¼ lean meat, 1 fat

■ ■ ■

Rigatoni with Broccoli Rabe & Ricotta

YIELD: 5 SERVINGS

8 ounces whole-wheat rigatoni or penne pasta

8 cups broccoli rabe, chopped into 1-inch
    pieces (about 12 ounces)

2 tablespoons extra virgin olive oil

1 ½ teaspoons crushed garlic

1 ½ cups diced fresh tomatoes

½ teaspoon salt

½ teaspoon coarsely ground black pepper

⅓ cup shredded Parmesan cheese

1 cup nonfat or light ricotta cheese

1. Cook the pasta al dente according to package directions. One minute before the pasta is done, add the broccoli rabe and cook for an additional minute, until the broccoli rabe is crisp-tender and the pasta is al dente. Drain well and set aside.

2. While the pasta is cooking, coat a large deep nonstick skillet with the olive oil and add the garlic. Cook over medium heat for about 15 seconds, just until the garlic begins to turn color and smells fragrant.

3. Add the tomatoes, salt, and pepper to the skillet, cover, and cook for a minute or two, until the tomatoes are heated through and start to soften.

4. Reduce the heat to low, add the pasta mixture to the skillet mixture, and toss to mix well. Serve hot, topping each serving with some of the Parmesan and a dollop of the ricotta cheese.

Nutritional Facts (per 1½-cup serving)

CALORIES: 313 CARBOHYDRATES: 42 g CHOLESTEROL: 7 mg
FAT: 8.3 g SAT. FAT: 2.1 g FIBER: 6.4 g PROTEIN: 18 g
SODIUM: 419 mg CALCIUM: 352 mg

Diabetic exchanges: 2½ starch, 1 vegetable, 1 lean meat, 1 fat

■ ■ ■

Penne with Italian Sausage & Broccoli Rabe

YIELD: 5 SERVINGS

8 ounces whole-wheat penne or rotini pasta

6 cups broccoli rabe, chopped into 1-inch pieces

1 pound hot or sweet turkey Italian sausage, casings removed

1 ½ teaspoons crushed garlic

14½-ounce can diced tomatoes with Italian seasonings

Grated Parmesan cheese (optional)

1. Cook the pasta al dente according to package directions. One minute before the pasta is done, add the broccoli rabe and cook for an additional minute, or until the broccoli rabe is crisp-tender and the pasta is al dente. Drain well and set aside.

2. While the pasta is cooking, coat a large, deep, nonstick skillet with nonstick cooking spray and add the sausage. Cook the sausage over medium heat, stirring to crumble, until the meat is no longer pink. Add the garlic and cook for a few seconds more.

3. Add the undrained tomatoes to the skillet mixture and cook for a minute or two, until heated through.

4. Reduce the heat to low, add the pasta mixture to the skillet mixture, and toss to mix well. Serve hot, topping each serving with some Parmesan cheese if desired.

Nutritional Facts (per 1¾-cup serving)
CALORIES: 348 CARBOHYDRATES: 42 g
CHOLESTEROL: 76 mg FAT: 9.2 g SAT. FAT: 2.6 g
FIBER: 4.9 g PROTEIN: 23 g SODIUM: 947 mg
CALCIUM: 57 mg
    Diabetic exchanges: 2½ starch, 1 vegetable, 2½ lean meat

▪ ▪ ▪

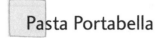

Pasta Portabella

YIELD: 4 SERVINGS

4 large portabella mushrooms, sliced ½-inch thick
Olive oil cooking spray
¼ teaspoon dried thyme
⅛ teaspoon ground black pepper
⅛ teaspoon salt
8 ounces whole-wheat penne pasta
2 cups marinara sauce, heated
½ cup shredded Parmesan cheese

1. Preheat oven to 450°.

2. Coat a large baking sheet with the cooking spray and lay the mushroom slices on the sheet. Spray the tops of the mushrooms lightly with the cooking spray and sprinkle with the thyme, pepper, and salt. Bake at 450 degrees for 10 minutes, turn the slices and bake for an additional 5 minutes, until the slices are tender and nicely browned. Remove the mushroom slices from the oven and set aside to keep warm.

3. While the mushrooms are cooking,

cook the pasta al dente according to package directions, drain well, and toss with the marinara sauce.

4. To serve, divide the pasta mixture between 4 serving dishes and top each serving with some of the mushroom slices and Parmesan cheese. Serve hot.

Nutritional Facts (per serving)
CALORIES: 306 CARBOHYDRATES: 52 g CHOLESTEROL: 7 mg
FAT: 3.9 g SAT. FAT: 1.9 g FIBER: 6.2 g PROTEIN: 14.5 g
SODIUM: 649 mg CALCIUM: 139 mg
    Diabetic exchanges: 3 starch, 1½ vegetable, ½ high-fat meat

▪ ▪ ▪

Tortellini Primavera

YIELD: 4 SERVINGS

12 ounces refrigerated reduced-fat cheese
    tortellini (about 3 cups)
1½ cups small broccoli florets
2 medium yellow squash, halved lengthwise and
    sliced (about 1¼ cups)
1¼ cups sliced fresh mushrooms
1 cup red bell pepper strips or sliced carrots
2½ cups ready-made marinara sauce, heated
¼ cup plus 2 tablespoons shredded
    Parmesan cheese

1. Cook the tortellini al dente according to package directions. Drain well, return to the pot, and cover to keep warm.

2. While the pasta is cooking, coat a large nonstick skillet with nonstick cooking spray or 1 tablespoon extra virgin olive oil and preheat over medium-high heat. Add the vegetables, cover, and cook, stirring frequently for about 4 minutes, until the vegetables are crisp-tender. Add a few teaspoons of water to the skillet if it becomes too dry.

3. Spread a quarter of the sauce over the bottom of each of 4 serving plates. Top the sauce on each plate with a quarter of the tortellini, leaving a 1-inch border of sauce showing under the pasta. Spoon a quarter of the vegetable mixture over the pasta and sprinkle with some of the Parmesan. Serve hot.

Nutritional Facts (per serving)
CALORIES: 381 CARBOHYDRATES: 53 g
CHOLESTEROL: 44 mg FAT: 10 g SAT. FAT: 5 g FIBER: 5.5 g
PROTEIN: 20 g SODIUM: 891 mg CALCIUM: 309 mg

Diabetic exchanges: 2½ starch, 3 vegetable, 1 high-fat meat

■ ■ ■

Pasta Pie with Broccoli & Italian Sausage

Similar to a frittata, this pasta pie is a great way to use up leftover pasta.

YIELD: 6 SERVINGS

12 ounces turkey Italian sausage, casings removed
1½ cups chopped fresh mushrooms

10-ounce package frozen chopped broccoli or spinach, thawed
1 teaspoon crushed garlic
2½ cups cooked thin spaghetti (about 5 ounces dry)
1¼ cups shredded reduced-fat mozzarella or provolone cheese
2 cups fat-free egg substitute
2 tablespoons grated Parmesan cheese
olive oil cooking spray

1. Preheat oven to 400°.

2. Coat a large nonstick skillet with cooking spray and place over medium heat. Add the sausage and cook for several minutes, stirring to crumble until the sausage is no longer pink. Add the mushrooms, broccoli or spinach, and garlic. Cover and cook for a few minutes more, until the vegetables are tender. Drain off any excess liquid.

3. Place the sausage and vegetables in a large bowl and toss in the spaghetti. Next toss in the mozzarella and egg substitute.

4. Respray the skillet with cooking spray and spread the pasta mixture evenly in the dish. Sprinkle the Parmesan cheese over the top and spray the top lightly with the cooking spray. Bake uncovered for about 20 minutes, until the center of the pie is set but still moist. Let sit for 5 minutes before cutting into wedges and serving.

Nutritional Facts (per serving)
CALORIES: 305 CARBOHYDRATES: 22 g
CHOLESTEROL: 62 mg FAT: 10 g SAT. FAT: 4.5 g

FIBER: 2 g PROTEIN: 30 g SODIUM: 745 mg CALCIUM: 305 mg

Diabetic exchanges: 1¼ starch, 1 vegetable, 3½ lean meat

■ ■ ■

Spaghetti with Sun-Dried Tomato Clam Sauce

YIELD: 5 SERVINGS

8 ounces whole-wheat thin spaghetti

2 cups sliced fresh mushrooms

1½ teaspoons crushed garlic

¾ teaspoon dried Italian seasoning

¼ teaspoon ground black pepper

2 cans (6 ounces each) chopped clams

½ cup plus 2 tablespoons julienne sun-dried
    tomatoes in olive oil and Italian seasonings,
    undrained

¼ cup finely chopped fresh parsley

⅓ cup grated Parmesan cheese
    (optional)

1. Cook the pasta al dente according to package directions. Drain, return to the pot, and cover to keep warm.

2. Coat a large nonstick skillet with cooking spray and place over medium-high heat. Add the mushrooms, garlic, Italian seasoning, and pepper, and sauté until the mushrooms are tender.

3. Add the juice from the clams to the skillet and bring to a boil. Cook over medium-high heat for several minutes, until the clam juice is reduced by half. Add the clams and undrained tomatoes to the skillet mixture and heat through. Add the spaghetti to the skillet mixture and toss to mix well.

4. Serve hot, topping each serving with some of the parsley and, if desired, some Parmesan cheese.

Nutritional Facts (per 1¼-cup serving)
CALORIES: 356 CARBOHYDRATES: 49 g
CHOLESTEROL: 24 mg FAT: 7.6 g SAT. FAT: 0.2 g
FIBER: 8.4 g PROTEIN: 20 g SODIUM: 191 mg
CALCIUM: 91 mg

Diabetic exchanges: 2½ starch, 1½ vegetable, 2 very lean meat, 1½ fat

■ ■ ■

Spicy Chicken Pie

For variety, substitute ¾ pound browned lean ground beef or a 15-ounce can of drained black beans for the chicken.

YIELD: 6 SERVINGS

CRUST

3 cups cooked orzo pasta (about 1 cup dry)

¼ cup plus 2 tablespoons grated Parmesan
    cheese

¼ cup fat-free egg substitute or 2 egg whites,
    lightly beaten

Butter-flavored cooking spray

1½ cups coarsely chopped fresh mushrooms

1 medium yellow onion, sliced and separated into rings

1½ cups shredded or diced roasted chicken

14½-ounce can Mexican-style stewed tomatoes, crushed

1½ teaspoons chili powder

1 cup shredded reduced-fat Monterey Jack or Mexican-blend cheese

1. Preheat oven to 375°.

2. To make the crust, place the orzo, Parmesan cheese, and egg substitute or egg whites in a large bowl and stir to mix well. Coat a 10-inch pie pan with the cooking spray and pat the mixture evenly over the bottom and sides of the pan, forming an even crust. Spray the crust lightly with the cooking spray and bake uncovered for 10 minutes.

3. While the crust is baking, coat a large nonstick skillet with nonstick cooking spray and add the mushrooms and onions. Place the skillet over medium heat, cover, and cook, stirring occasionally, for several minutes until the vegetables are tender. Add the undrained tomatoes, chili powder, and chicken to the skillet mixture. Cook uncovered, stirring occasionally, for about 5 minutes, until the mixture is thick.

4. Spoon the chicken mixture into the baked crust and sprinkle the cheese over the top. Bake for an additional 5 minutes or until the cheese is melted. Cut into wedges and serve hot.

Nutritional Facts (per serving)

CALORIES: 295 CARBOHYDRATES: 29 g
CHOLESTEROL: 46 mg FAT: 7.7 g SAT. FAT: 3.3 g
FIBER: 2 g PROTEIN: 25 g SODIUM: 426 mg
CALCIUM: 297 mg

Diabetic exchanges: 1½ starch, 2½ lean meat, 1 vegetable

■ ■ ■

Lazy-Day Lasagna

YIELD: 8 SERVINGS

¾ pound 95% lean ground beef or turkey Italian sausage

1 cup chopped onion

26-ounce jar marinara sauce

14½-ounce can diced Italian-style or roasted garlic tomatoes

10 uncooked whole-wheat lasagna noodles (about 8 ounces)

2 cups shredded nonfat or reduced-fat mozzarella cheese

¼ cup grated Parmesan cheese

CHEESE FILLING

15 ounces nonfat or part-skim ricotta cheese

3 tablespoons fat-free egg substitute

1 teaspoon dried parsley

1. Preheat oven to 350°.

2. Coat a large nonstick skillet with nonstick cooking spray and add the ground beef or sausage. Cook over medium heat, stirring

to crumble until the meat is no longer pink. Drain off and discard any fat. Add the onions and cook for several minutes, until the onions are tender. Stir in the marinara sauce and undrained tomatoes and cook for another minute or two to heat through. Cover the sauce to keep warm and set aside.

3. To make the cheese filling, place all of the cheese filling ingredients in a medium-sized bowl and stir to mix well. Set aside.

4. To assemble the lasagna, coat a 9 × 13-inch baking pan with nonstick cooking spray and spoon 1½ cups of the sauce over the bottom of the pan. Lay 5 of the uncooked noodles over the sauce to cover the bottom of the pan, arranging 4 of the noodles lengthwise, slightly overlapping, and 1 noodle crosswise. (You will have to break about 1 inch off the bottom of the crosswise noodle to make it fit in the pan.)

5. Spread all of the cheese filling over the noodles, then top with half of the mozzarella, and another 1½ cups of sauce. Finish layering the casserole with the remaining noodles, sauce, and mozzarella. Sprinkle the Parmesan over the top.

6. Place the casserole on a large baking sheet (to catch any drips), cover the pan with aluminum foil (spray the underside of the foil with cooking spray to prevent sticking), and bake* for 45 minutes. Remove the foil and bake for an additional 15 minutes, until hot and bubbly and lightly browned on top. Let stand for 20 minutes before cutting into squares and serving.

Nutritional Facts (per serving)
CALORIES: 356 CARBOHYDRATES: 34 g
CHOLESTEROL: 45 mg FAT: 9 g SAT. FAT: 5 g FIBER: 3.5 g
PROTEIN: 33 g SODIUM: 621 mg CALCIUM: 553 mg
    Diabetic exchanges: 2 starch, 1½ vegetable, 3 lean meat

*This casserole can be assembled ahead of time and refrigerated for up to twenty-four hours before baking. Let the dish sit at room temperature for 30 to 60 minutes before placing in the oven.

■ ■ ■

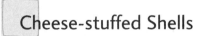

Cheese-stuffed Shells

YIELD: 6 SERVINGS

18 jumbo pasta shells (about 4½ ounces)
¾ cup shredded reduced-fat mozzarella cheese

SAUCE
14½-ounce can diced tomatoes with Italian
    seasonings or roasted garlic
3 tablespoons tomato paste with Italian
    seasonings or roasted garlic

FILLING
15 ounces nonfat or light ricotta cheese
1 cup nonfat or low-fat cottage cheese
¾ cup shredded reduced-fat mozzarella cheese
¼ cup grated Parmesan cheese
¼ cup fat-free egg substitute
2 teaspoons dried parsley

1. Preheat oven to 350°.

2. Cook the pasta al dente according to package directions. Drain, rinse with cool water, and drain again. Set aside.

3. To make the sauce, place the undrained tomatoes and tomato paste in a 1-quart pot and stir to mix well. Cover and cook over medium heat for several minutes, until heated through. Set aside to keep warm.

4. Place all of the filling ingredients in a medium-sized bowl and stir to mix well. Set aside.

5. To assemble the dish, coat a 9 × 13-inch baking pan with nonstick cooking spray and spread a thin layer of the sauce over the bottom of the pan. Spoon a heaping tablespoon of filling into each shell and arrange the stuffed shells in a single layer in the prepared pan. Pour the remaining sauce over the shells.

6. Cover the dish with aluminum foil and bake for 25 minutes, until heated through. Sprinkle the mozzarella cheese over the top and bake uncovered for an additional 5 minutes, until the cheese is melted. Remove the dish from the oven and let sit for 5 minutes before serving.

Nutritional Facts (per serving)
CALORIES: 309 CARBOHYDRATES: 30 g
CHOLESTEROL: 24 mg FAT: 6.5 g SAT. FAT: 3.9 g
FIBER: 1.7 g PROTEIN: 31 g SODIUM: 770 mg
CALCIUM: 671 mg
   Diabetic exchanges: 1½ starch, 1 vegetable, 2½ lean meat

■ ■ ■

Baked Ziti with Roasted Chicken & Red Peppers

YIELD: 6 SERVINGS

8 ounces whole-wheat ziti or penne pasta
2 cups sliced fresh mushrooms
26-ounce jar marinara sauce (about 3 cups)
12-ounce jar roasted red bell peppers, drained and chopped (about 1 cup)
¼ to ½ teaspoon crushed red pepper
2½ cups shredded or diced roasted skinless rotisserie chicken
¼ cup grated Parmesan cheese
1¼ cups shredded reduced-fat mozzarella or provolone cheese

1. Preheat oven to 375°.

2. Cook the pasta according to package directions, drain, and return to the pot.

3. Coat a large, deep, nonstick skillet with cooking spray and add the mushrooms. Cook over medium heat for several minutes, until the mushrooms are tender. Stir in the sauce, roasted red peppers, and crushed red pepper and cook for another minute or two, until heated through.

4. Add the sauce mixture, chicken, and half of the Parmesan cheese to the pasta and toss to mix well. Coat a 9 × 13-inch pan with nonstick cooking spray and spread the pasta mixture evenly in the pan. Sprinkle the remaining Parmesan cheese over the top.

5. Cover the pan with aluminum foil (spray the underside of the foil with cooking spray to prevent sticking) and bake for 20 minutes, until heated through. Remove the foil and top with the mozzarella cheese. Bake for an additional 5 minutes, until the cheese is melted. Serve hot.

Nutritional Facts (per 1⅔-cup serving)
CALORIES: 379 CARBOHYDRATES: 39 g
CHOLESTEROL: 66 mg FAT: 8.2 g SAT. FAT: 4.1 g
FIBER: 5 g PROTEIN: 34 g SODIUM: 641 mg
CALCIUM: 249 mg
  Diabetic exchanges: 2 starch, 1½ vegetable, 3 lean meat

▨ ▨ ▨

15. LIGHT AND EASY ENTRÉES

Many people believe that adopting a diabetes prevention diet means spending hours in the kitchen preparing complicated recipes and perusing specialty stores for exotic and expensive ingredients. As you will see, nothing could be further from the truth. This chapter will prove that light and delicious meals can be easily prepared using ingredients that are available in your local grocery store.

As you glance through these pages, remember that these are just some of the savory dishes that are within your reach. Delicious pasta entrées can be found in chapter 14, a wide variety of main dish salads can be found in chapter 11, and hearty soups are featured in chapter 10. And for a change of pace, try having breakfast for dinner—chapter 8 presents many delicious possibilities.

When planning your diabetes-fighting meals, remember to balance your entrée with the appropriate side dishes. For instance, if you are having a starch-based entrée like Spicy Chicken Enchiladas, pair it with a fresh garden salad and a low-carbohydrate vegetable like sautéed zucchini or green beans with almonds. Add other starches like rice only if you need the extra carbohydrates and calories.

Stuffed Chicken Breast Florentine

YIELD: 4 SERVINGS

4 cups (packed) coarsely chopped fresh spinach

2 teaspoons crushed garlic

¼ cup crumbled reduced-fat feta cheese (plain or flavored with tomatoes and basil)

4 boneless skinless chicken breast halves (5 ounces each)

1 tablespoon extra virgin olive oil

½ teaspoon salt

½ teaspoon ground black pepper

1. Coat a large skillet with nonstick cooking spray. Add the spinach and garlic and cook for a couple of minutes over medium heat, until the spinach is wilted. Remove from the heat and toss in the feta cheese.

2. Cut a deep pocket into the thickest side of each piece of chicken and stuff a quarter of the spinach mixture into each pocket. Close by pressing the flesh together and secure with a wooden toothpick if necessary. Sprinkle both sides of the chicken pieces with some of the salt and pepper.

3. Wipe out the skillet, add the olive oil, and preheat over medium-high heat. Add the chicken and cook for a couple of minutes on each side, until nicely browned. Reduce the heat to medium-low, cover, and cook for about 8 to 10 minutes, turning occasionally, until the chicken is cooked through. Serve hot.

Nutritional Facts (per serving)

CALORIES: 213 CARBOHYDRATES: 2 g CHOLESTEROL: 84 mg FAT: 6.7 g SAT. FAT: 1.6 g FIBER: 1 g PROTEIN: 35 g SODIUM: 525 mg CALCIUM: 92 mg

Diabetic exchanges: 3 very lean meat, 1 vegetable, ½ fat

▪ ▪ ▪

Tarragon Chicken & Mushrooms

YIELD: 4 SERVINGS

1 teaspoon dried tarragon

½ teaspoon garlic powder

½ teaspoon ground black pepper

¼ teaspoon salt

1 pound boneless skinless chicken breast, cut into 8 equal pieces and pounded ¼-inch thick

1 tablespoon extra virgin olive oil

3 cups sliced fresh mushrooms

½ cup chicken broth

1. Combine the tarragon, garlic powder, pepper, and salt and sprinkle both sides of the chicken pieces with some of the seasoning.

2. Coat a large nonstick skillet with the olive oil and preheat over medium-high heat. Add the chicken and cook for a couple of

minutes on each side, until nicely browned and cooked through. Remove the chicken from the skillet and set aside to keep warm.

3. Add the mushrooms to the skillet and sauté for a couple of minutes, until tender. Add the broth and cook uncovered for several minutes, until only a couple of tablespoons of liquid remain.

4. To serve, place 2 pieces of chicken on each of 4 serving plates and top with some of the mushrooms and pan juices. Serve hot.

Nutritional Facts (per serving)

CALORIES: 161 CARBOHYDRATES: 3 g CHOLESTEROL: 66 mg FAT: 3.9 g SAT. FAT: 1 g FIBER: 0.8 g PROTEIN: 28 g SODIUM: 324 mg CALCIUM: 20 mg

   Diabetic exchanges: 3 very lean meat, 1 vegetable, ½ fat

■ ■ ■

Apricot-Ginger Chicken

YIELD: 4 SERVINGS

SAUCE

¼ cup plus 2 tablespoons low-sodium chicken
   broth
¼ cup light (reduced-sugar) apricot fruit spread
1 tablespoon rice vinegar
1 tablespoon reduced-sodium soy sauce
½ teaspoon ground ginger

¼ teaspoon garlic powder
¼ teaspoon ground black pepper

¼ teaspoon salt
1 pound boneless skinless chicken breast, cut
   into 8 equal pieces and pounded ¼-inch thick
1 tablespoon canola oil
3 tablespoons thinly sliced scallions

1. Place all of the sauce ingredients in a medium bowl and stir to mix well. Set aside.

2. Combine the garlic powder, pepper, and salt and sprinkle both sides of the chicken pieces with some of the seasoning.

3. Place the oil in a large nonstick skillet and preheat over medium-high heat. Add the chicken and cook for a couple of minutes on each side, until nicely browned and no longer pink inside. Remove the chicken from the skillet and set aside to keep warm.

4. Pour the sauce into the skillet and cook, stirring frequently, for a couple of minutes, or until sauce is reduced by almost half and is syrupy.

5. To serve, place 2 pieces of chicken on each of 4 serving plates. Drizzle each serving with some of the sauce and top with a sprinkling of scallions. Serve hot.

Nutritional Facts (per serving)

CALORIES: 176 CARBOHYDRATES: 6 g CHOLESTEROL: 66 mg FAT: 4.8 g SAT. FAT: 0.6 g FIBER: 0.1 g PROTEIN: 26 g SODIUM: 445 mg CALCIUM: 16 mg

   Diabetic exchanges: 3 very lean meat, ⅓ other carbohydrate, ½ fat

■ ■ ■

utes. Add the raisins and simmer for an additional 5 minutes.

3. Serve hot over brown rice or whole-wheat couscous if desired. Top each serving with a sprinkling of almonds and parsley.

Nutritional Facts (per serving)

CALORIES: 268 CARBOHYDRATES: 19 g
CHOLESTEROL: 66 mg FAT: 8.6 g SAT. FAT: 0.9 g
FIBER: 3.2 g PROTEIN: 29 g SODIUM: 446 mg
CALCIUM: 74 mg

 Diabetic exchanges: 3 very lean meat, 1½ vegetable, ½ fruit, 1 fat

■ ■ ■

Quick Curried Chicken

YIELD: 4 SERVINGS

1 tablespoon canola oil
1 pound boneless skinless chicken breast, cut into bite-size pieces
½ teaspoon dried thyme
¼ teaspoon salt
¼ teaspoon ground black pepper
1 medium yellow onion, chopped
1 medium green bell pepper, chopped
1 14½-ounce can stewed tomatoes, crushed
1 to 2 teaspoons curry paste or curry powder, or more to taste
¼ cup dark raisins
¼ cup sliced almonds
2 tablespoons finely chopped fresh parsley or 2 teaspoons dried parsley, finely crumbled

1. Coat the bottom of a large nonstick skillet with the oil and preheat over medium-high heat. Add the chicken and sprinkle with the thyme, salt, and pepper. Cook, stirring frequently for several minutes, until the chicken is nicely browned.

2. Add the onions and peppers to the skillet. Cover and cook over medium heat for about 3 minutes, until the vegetables start to soften. Add the undrained tomatoes and curry to the skillet mixture and bring the mixture to a boil. Reduce the heat to low, cover, and cook, stirring occasionally, for 10 min-

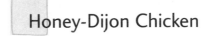

Honey-Dijon Chicken

YIELD: 4 SERVINGS

¾ teaspoon fines herbes or herbes de Provence
¼ teaspoon garlic powder
¼ teaspoon salt
¼ teaspoon ground black pepper
1 pound chicken tenders or 1 pound boneless skinless chicken breast, cut into 8 equal pieces and pounded ½-inch thick
1 tablespoon extra virgin olive oil
3 tablespoons thinly sliced scallions or finely chopped parsley

SAUCE
¼ cup plus 2 tablespoons chicken broth
1 tablespoon lemon juice
1 tablespoon Dijon mustard
1 tablespoon honey

1. Combine the herbs, garlic powder, salt, and pepper and sprinkle some of the mixture over both sides of the chicken pieces.

2. Coat a large nonstick skillet with the olive oil and preheat over medium-high heat. Add the chicken and cook for 2 minutes on each side, until nicely browned. Cover the skillet and reduce the heat to medium. Cook for about 3 minutes, turning once, until the chicken is cooked through. Remove the chicken from the skillet and set aside to keep warm.

3. Combine the sauce ingredients in a small bowl and stir to mix. Add the sauce to the skillet and bring the mixture to a boil over medium-high heat. Cook for a minute or 2, stirring frequently, until reduced by half.

4. To serve, place 2 chicken pieces on each of 4 serving plates, drizzle with some of the sauce, and top with a sprinkling of scallions or parsley. Serve hot.

Nutritional Facts (per serving)
CALORIES: 198 CARBOHYDRATES: 6 g
CHOLESTEROL: 66 mg FAT: 5.1 g SAT. FAT: 0.9 g
FIBER: 0.2 g PROTEIN: 26 g SODIUM: 367 mg
CALCIUM: 22 mg
   Diabetic exchanges: 3 very lean meat, ⅓ other carbohydrate, ½ fat

◼ ◼ ◼

Chicken Olé

YIELD: 4 SERVINGS

1 pound boneless skinless chicken breast, cut
   into bite-size pieces
1 teaspoon ground cumin
¼ teaspoon ground black pepper
1 tablespoon extra virgin olive oil
1 medium yellow onion, sliced and separated
   into rings
14½-ounce can Mexican-style stewed tomatoes
1 cup frozen (thawed) whole kernel corn
¼ cup chopped fresh cilantro or sliced scallions

1. Sprinkle the chicken with the cumin and pepper and toss to mix well. Set aside.

2. Coat a large nonstick skillet with the olive oil and preheat over medium-high heat. Add the chicken and cook for several minutes, until nicely browned. Add the onions, reduce the heat to medium, cover, and cook for a couple of minutes, until the onion softens.

3. Add the undrained tomatoes to the skillet and let the mixture come to a boil. Reduce the heat to low, cover, and cook for 10 minutes. Add the corn and cook covered for 5 minutes more. Serve hot, topping each serving with a sprinkling of the cilantro or scallions. Serve over brown rice or whole-wheat couscous if desired.

Nutritional Facts (per serving)
CALORIES: 231 CARBOHYDRATES: 18 g
CHOLESTEROL: 65 mg FAT: 5.2 g SAT. FAT: 0.9 g
FIBER: 3.2 g PROTEIN: 29 g SODIUM: 403 mg
CALCIUM: 38 mg
Diabetic exchanges: 3 very lean meat, ½ starch,
1½ vegetable, ½ fat

■ ■ ■

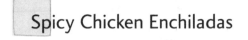

Spicy Chicken Enchiladas

YIELD: 4 SERVINGS

FILLING

1 ½ cups shredded skinless roasted chicken
4-ounce can chopped green chilies
¼ cup nonfat or light sour cream
¾ teaspoon ground cumin

8 thin corn tortillas (6-inch rounds)
1 ¾ cups canned enchilada sauce, heated
1 cup shredded reduced-fat Monterey Jack or
    Mexican-blend cheese

TOPPINGS

½ cup nonfat or light sour cream
¼ cup finely chopped scallions or fresh cilantro

1. Preheat oven to 450°.
2. Combine all of the filling ingredients in a bowl and toss to mix well. Set aside.
3. Coat a large nonstick skillet with cooking spray and preheat over medium heat. Place a tortilla in the pan and heat for 10 to 15 seconds on each side, until the tortilla is pliable enough to roll up.

4. Lay the tortilla on a flat surface and spread ¼ cup of the filling along one end. Roll the tortilla up to enclose the filling. Coat a 9 × 13-inch pan with nonstick cooking spray and lay the enchilada in the pan, seam side down. Repeat with the remaining tortillas, leaving a ¼-inch space between the enchiladas to prevent them from sticking together.

5. Pour the sauce over the enchiladas, covering them completely. Bake uncovered for 8 minutes. Sprinkle the cheese over the top and bake for about 3 minutes more, or until the cheese is melted.

6. Serve hot, topping each serving with some of the sour cream and scallions or cilantro.

Nutritional Facts (per serving)
CALORIES: 356 CARBOHYDRATES: 33 g CHOLESTEROL: 60
mg FAT: 9 g SAT. FAT: 2.7 g FIBER: 2.4 g PROTEIN: 30 g
SODIUM: 681 mg CALCIUM: 379 mg
Diabetic exchanges: 3 lean meat, 2 starch, ½ vegetable

■ ■ ■

Caribbean Chicken with Mango Salsa

YIELD: 4 SERVINGS

MANGO SALSA

1 cup ¼-inch diced fresh mango
¼ cup finely chopped green bell pepper

¼ cup finely chopped red bell pepper

¼ cup thinly sliced scallions

1 to 2 teaspoons finely chopped pickled
jalapeño peppers

2 teaspoons lime juice

⅛ teaspoon salt

1 pound chicken tenders or 1 pound boneless
skinless chicken breast cut into 8 equal pieces
and pounded ½-inch thick

1 tablespoon jerk seasoning

1 tablespoon plus 1 teaspoon extra virgin olive oil

1. Just before you are ready to cook the chicken, combine all of the salsa ingredients and stir to mix well. Set aside.

2. Rinse the chicken and pat dry with paper towels. Rub some of the jerk seasoning over all sides of the chicken.

3. Place the olive oil in a large nonstick skillet and preheat over medium-high heat. Add the chicken and cook for a couple of minutes on each side, until nicely browned. Reduce the heat to medium, cover, and cook for about 3 minutes more, until the chicken is cooked through.

4. Divide the chicken among 4 serving plates and serve hot, accompanied by the salsa.

Nutritional Facts (per serving)
CALORIES: 202 CARBOHYDRATES: 9 g CHOLESTEROL: 66 mg
FAT: 6 g SAT. FAT: 1 g FIBER: 1.3 g PROTEIN: 27 g
SODIUM: 514 mg CALCIUM: 19 mg
Diabetic exchanges: 3 very lean meat, ½ fruit, 1 fat

■ ■ ■

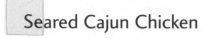

Seared Cajun Chicken

YIELD: 4 SERVINGS

1 pound chicken tenders or 1 pound boneless
skinless chicken breast cut into 8 equal pieces
and pounded ½-inch thick

1 tablespoon Cajun seasoning

1 tablespoon extra virgin olive oil

½ cup chicken broth

2 tablespoons finely chopped fresh parsley or 2
teaspoons dried parsley, finely crumbled

1. Rinse the chicken and pat dry with paper towels. Rub some of the Cajun seasoning over both sides of the chicken pieces.

2. Coat a large nonstick skillet with the olive oil and preheat over medium-high heat. Add the chicken and cook for a couple of minutes on each side, until nicely browned. Cover the skillet and reduce the heat to medium. Cook for about 3 minutes, turning once, until the chicken is thoroughly cooked. Remove the chicken from the skillet and set aside to keep warm.

3. Add the broth to the skillet and cook over medium-high heat for several minutes or until reduced to about 3 tablespoons in volume.

4. To serve, divide the chicken among 4 serving plates, drizzle with some of the sauce and top with a sprinkling of parsley. Serve hot.

Nutritional Facts (per serving)
CALORIES: 160 CARBOHYDRATES: 1 g
CHOLESTEROL: 66 mg FAT: 4.9 g SAT. FAT: 0.8 g
FIBER: 0.2 g PROTEIN: 26 g SODIUM: 470 mg
CALCIUM: 15 mg
   Diabetic exchanges: 3 very lean meat, 1 fat

■ ■ ■

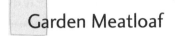# Garden Meatloaf

YIELD: 6 SERVINGS

1½ pounds 95% lean ground beef
¾ cup quick-cooking oats
¾ cup finely chopped onion
½ cup finely chopped green bell pepper
½ cup grated carrot
½ cup vegetable juice cocktail (like V8)
¼ cup plus 2 tablespoons fat-free egg substitute
1½ teaspoons crushed garlic or ³⁄₈ teaspoon
   garlic powder
2 teaspoons dried parsley, finely crumbled
1 teaspoon dried thyme or marjoram
½ teaspoon ground black pepper
¼ teaspoon salt
½ cup ketchup

1. Preheat oven to 350°.
2. Place all of the ingredients except the ketchup in a large bowl and mix well. Coat a 9 × 5-inch meatloaf pan with cooking spray and press the mixture into the pan to form a loaf.

3. Bake uncovered for 45 minutes. Spread the ketchup over the meat loaf and bake for 30 additional minutes, or until the meat is no longer pink inside and a meat thermometer reads at least 160 degrees.

4. Remove the loaf from the oven and let it sit for 10 minutes before slicing and serving.

Nutritional Facts (per serving)
CALORIES: 228 CARBOHYDRATES: 17 g
CHOLESTEROL: 60 mg FAT: 5.8 g SAT. FAT: 2.2 g
FIBER: 2.3 g PROTEIN: 26 g SODIUM: 406 mg
CALCIUM: 27 mg
   Diabetic exchanges: 3 lean meat, ½ vegetable, 1 starch

■ ■ ■

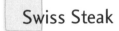# Swiss Steak

YIELD: 4 SERVINGS

1 pound well-trimmed beef top round steak
   (about ¾-inch thick), cut into 8 equal pieces
2 tablespoons whole-wheat pastry flour or
   unbleached flour
½ teaspoon ground black pepper
1 tablespoon canola oil
1 medium yellow onion, sliced and separated
   into rings
14½-ounce can stewed tomatoes

1. Rinse the meat and pat dry with paper towels. Combine the flour and pepper and, using a meat mallet, pound the flour mixture

into the meat until the meat is slightly less than ½-inch thick.

2. Coat a large nonstick skillet with the oil and preheat over medium-high heat. Add the steak pieces and cook for a couple of minutes on each side, until nicely browned. Top with the onions and pour the undrained tomatoes over the top.

3. Cover and cook over low heat for about 45 minutes, until the meat is tender. Serve hot.

Nutritional Facts (per serving)

CALORIES: 257 CARBOHYDRATES: 12 g
CHOLESTEROL: 76 mg FAT: 8.5 g SAT. FAT: 2 g
FIBER: 1.6 g PROTEIN: 32 g SODIUM: 266 mg
CALCIUM: 43 mg

Diabetic exchanges: 3 lean meat, 1 vegetable, ½ starch, ½ fat

◼ ◼ ◼

Meat & Potato Pie

YIELD: 5 SERVINGS

TOPPING

1 pound Yukon Gold potatoes (about 3 medium)
½ cup nonfat or light sour cream
¼ teaspoon salt
Pinch ground white pepper
Butter-flavored cooking spray
Ground paprika

1 pound 95% lean ground beef
½ cup chopped onion
¾ cup water
10-ounce package frozen mixed vegetables
10¾-ounce can condensed golden mushroom soup, undiluted

1. Preheat oven to 350°.

2. To make the topping, peel the potatoes and cut them into 1-inch pieces (there should be about 3 cups). Place the potatoes in a 2½-quart pot, barely cover with water, and bring to a boil. Reduce the heat to medium, cover, and cook for 10 minutes, until the potatoes are soft.

3. Drain the potatoes, reserving ½ cup of the water. Add the sour cream, salt, pepper, and half of the reserved water and mash the potatoes with a potato masher until smooth. If the potatoes are too stiff, add a little more of the reserved water. Cover and set aside to keep warm.

4. While the potatoes are cooking, place the meat in a large nonstick ovenproof skillet and cook over medium heat, stirring to crumble, until the meat is no longer pink. Stir in the onions, cover, and cook for a couple of minutes, or until the onions begin to soften.

5. Add the water and the mixed vegetables to the skillet and stir to separate the vegetables. Cover and cook over medium-high heat for about 5 minutes, stirring occasionally, until the vegetables are barely tender. Add the undiluted soup to the skillet, and stir

to mix well. Cook, stirring occasionally for a minute or two, just until the mixture comes to a boil. Remove the skillet from the heat.

6. Drop the potatoes in 5 mounds over the skillet mixture. Spray the tops of the potatoes with the cooking spray and sprinkle lightly with the paprika. Bake at 350 degrees for about 25 minutes, until bubbly around the edges. Serve hot.

Nutritional Facts (per serving)
CALORIES: 280 CARBOHYDRATES: 32 g
CHOLESTEROL: 51 mg FAT: 5.9 g SAT. FAT: 2.2 g
FIBER: 4.3 g PROTEIN: 24 g SODIUM: 659 mg
CALCIUM: 51 mg
  Diabetic exchanges: 2½ lean meat, 1 vegetable, 1½ starch

■ ■ ■

Slow-cooked Sicilian Pot Roast

YIELD: 8 SERVINGS

2½-pound well-trimmed top round roast or flat half brisket
½ teaspoon coarsely ground black pepper
2 cups sliced fresh mushrooms
1 cup chopped onions
1 cup chopped red or green bell peppers or 1 cup roasted red bell peppers, drained and chopped

14½-ounce can diced Italian-style tomatoes, undrained
6-ounce can tomato paste with roasted garlic or Italian seasonings

1. Rinse the meat with cool water and pat it dry with paper towels. Sprinkle both sides with some of the pepper. Coat a large nonstick skillet with nonstick cooking spray and preheat over medium-high heat. Place the meat in the skillet and cook for 2 to 3 minutes on each side, until nicely browned.

2. Place the mushrooms, onions, and bell peppers in a 3-quart slow cooker and top with the roast. Pour the tomatoes over the meat. Cover and cook on high for 5 hours or on low for 10 hours, until the meat is very tender.

3. Remove the roast to a serving platter and cover loosely with aluminum foil to keep warm. Add the tomato paste to the remaining slow cooker mixture and stir to mix well.

4. Slice the roast across the grain and serve hot accompanied by the sauce. Serve with pasta if desired.

Nutritional Facts (per serving)
CALORIES: 221 CARBOHYDRATES: 12 g
CHOLESTEROL: 80 mg FAT: 5.7 g SAT. FAT: 1.7 g
FIBER: 2 g PROTEIN: 29 g SODIUM: 440 mg
CALCIUM: 36 mg
  Diabetic exchanges: 3 lean meat, 2 vegetable

■ ■ ■

Pork Tenderloin with Butternut Squash & Onions

YIELD: 4 SERVINGS

1 pound pork tenderloin (about 1 large)

3 cups 1-inch chunks diced peeled butternut squash or sweet potatoes

1 tablespoon extra virgin olive oil

1 teaspoon dried rosemary or fines herbes

½ teaspoon salt

¼ teaspoon ground black pepper

2 medium-small yellow onions, sliced ¼-inch thick and separated into rings

1. Preheat oven to 400°.

2. Rinse the pork with cool water and pat dry with paper towels. Coat a 9 × 13-inch pan with cooking spray and lay the tenderloin in the pan.

3. Place the squash and olive oil in a bowl and toss to mix well. Arrange the squash around the pork. Sprinkle the pork and squash with the herbs, salt, and pepper.

4. Bake for 10 minutes. Stir the onions into the squash and bake for an additional 20 minutes, stirring the vegetable mixture a couple of times, until a meat thermometer inserted in the thickest part of the pork reads 155 to 160 degrees and the squash mixture is tender and nicely browned.

5. Remove the pan from the oven, cover loosely with aluminum foil, and let sit for 5 minutes before slicing the pork thinly at an angle and serving.

Nutritional Facts (per serving)
CALORIES: 234 CARBOHYDRATES: 16 g
CHOLESTEROL: 67 mg FAT: 7.8 g SAT. FAT: 1.9 g
FIBER: 4.6 g PROTEIN: 26 g SODIUM: 344 mg
CALCIUM: 237 mg
Diabetic exchanges: 3 lean meat, 1 starch, ½ fat

■ ■ ■

Pork Medallions with Apple-Apricot Chutney

For variety, substitute golden raisins or dried cranberries for the dried apricots.

YIELD: 4 SERVINGS

1 pound pork tenderloin, cut into 8 equal pieces and pounded ¼-inch thick

¼ teaspoon salt

½ teaspoon coarsely ground black pepper

1 tablespoon extra virgin olive oil

3 tablespoons thinly sliced scallions

CHUTNEY

¾ cup diced yellow onion

1¼ cups chopped peeled Granny Smith apples (about 2 medium)

¼ cup plus 2 tablespoons chopped dried apricots

1 tablespoon apple cider vinegar

¾ teaspoon ground ginger

½ teaspoon dry mustard

½ cup plus 2 tablespoons apple juice

1. Sprinkle both sides of the pork pieces with some of the salt and pepper. Set aside.

2. To make the chutney, coat a large nonstick skillet with nonstick cooking spray and add the onion. Cover and cook over medium heat for about 3 minutes, until the onion starts to soften (add a little water if the skillet becomes too dry). Add the apples, apricots, vinegar, ginger, mustard, and about ⅓ cup of the apple juice. Cover and cook over medium heat for about 5 minutes, stirring occasionally, until the apples and onions are tender and the apricots are plumped. Remove the mixture from the skillet and set aside.

3. Wipe out the skillet, and then coat with the olive oil and preheat over medium-high heat. Add the pork and cook for 2 to 3 minutes on each side, until nicely browned and no longer pink inside. Remove the pork from the skillet and set aside to keep warm.

4. Return the apple mixture to the skillet and add the remaining apple juice. Bring the mixture to a boil over medium-high heat and cook for a couple of minutes, stirring frequently, until most of the liquid has evaporated.

5. To serve, place 2 pork medallions on each of 4 serving plates and top with some of the chutney and a sprinkling of scallions. Serve hot.

Nutritional Facts (per serving)

CALORIES: 231 CARBOHYDRATES: 20 g

CHOLESTEROL: 76 mg FAT: 6.2 g SAT. FAT: 1.5 g

FIBER: 2.5 g PROTEIN: 25 g SODIUM: 207 mg

CALCIUM: 19 mg

Diabetic exchanges: 3 lean meat, 1 fruit, ½ fat

▪ ▪ ▪

Pork Chops with Mushrooms & Onions

YIELD: 4 SERVINGS

4 well-trimmed pork loin chops (4 ounces each)

¾ teaspoon dried thyme

½ teaspoon garlic powder

½ teaspoon coarsely ground black pepper

Scant ½ teaspoon salt

2½ cups sliced mushrooms

1 medium yellow onion, sliced and separated into rings

1 tablespoon extra virgin olive oil

2 tablespoons dry sherry

1. Rinse the chops with cool water and pat dry with paper towels. Combine the thyme, garlic, pepper, and salt, and sprinkle some of the mixture over both sides of each pork chop. Set aside.

2. Coat a large nonstick skillet with cooking spray and add the mushrooms and onions. Place the skillet over medium-high heat. Cover and cook for a couple of minutes,

until the vegetables start to soften. Reduce the heat to medium and cook for several minutes more, until the vegetables are tender. Transfer the vegetables to a small dish and set aside to keep warm.

3. Wipe out the skillet, add the olive oil, and preheat over medium-high heat. Cook the pork chops for a couple of minutes on each side, until nicely browned. Reduce the heat to medium-low, cover, and cook for about 8 minutes, turning occasionally, until they are cooked through. Remove from the skillet and set aside to keep warm.

4. Add the sherry to the pan juices in the skillet and cook uncovered for about 1 minute, until reduced by half. Place the vegetables back in the skillet and toss in the pan juices for a minute or two, until most of the liquid has evaporated.

5. To serve, place 1 pork chop on each of 4 serving plates and top with some of the vegetable mixture. Serve hot.

Nutritional Facts (per serving)

CALORIES: 191 CARBOHYDRATES: 4 g CHOLESTEROL: 58 mg FAT: 8.3 g SAT. FAT: 2.3 g FIBER: 1.2 g PROTEIN: 23 g SODIUM: 278 mg CALCIUM: 30 mg

Diabetic exchanges: 3 lean meat, 1 vegetable, ½ fat

■ ■ ■

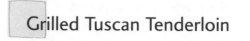

Grilled Tuscan Tenderloin

YIELD: 8 SERVINGS

MARINADE

½ cup orange juice

3 tablespoons balsamic vinegar

2 tablespoons extra virgin olive oil

2 tablespoons honey or brown sugar

2 teaspoons crushed garlic

2 teaspoons dried rosemary

1 teaspoon dried thyme or sage

1 teaspoon coarsely ground black pepper

1 teaspoon salt

2 pork tenderloins (1 pound each)

1. Combine all of the marinade ingredients in a bowl and stir to mix. Remove a ¼ cup of the marinade and refrigerate until ready to cook the tenderloins.

2. Place the tenderloins in a shallow nonmetal container. Pour the remaining marinade over the tenderloins and lift the meat to allow the marinade to flow underneath. Cover and refrigerate for 6 to 24 hours, turning occasionally.

3. Coat a grill rack with cooking spray and place the tenderloins on the grill rack. Cook, covered, over medium coals, turning occasionally, for about 20 minutes, until a thermometer inserted in the thickest part of

the meat reads 155 to 160 degrees. Baste occasionally with the reserved marinade during the last 5 minutes of cooking.

3. Remove the tenderloins from the grill, cover loosely with foil, and let sit for 5 minutes before slicing thinly at an angle and serving.

Nutritional Facts (per 3-ounce serving)
CALORIES: 166 CARBOHYDRATES: 3 g
CHOLESTEROL: 67 mg FAT: 5 g SAT. FAT: 1.6 g
FIBER: 0 g PROTEIN: 24 g SODIUM: 121 mg
CALCIUM: 8 mg
   Diabetic exchanges: 3 lean meat

▪ ▪ ▪

Scallops with Peanut Sauce

YIELD: 4 SERVINGS

SAUCE
¾ cup orange juice
¼ cup reduced-sodium Teriyaki sauce
2 to 3 tablespoons creamy peanut butter
½ teaspoon ground ginger

1¼ pounds large scallops, rinsed and patted dry
1 tablespoon canola oil
2 tablespoons thinly sliced scallions
2 tablespoons finely chopped fresh cilantro
   or parsley

1. Place all of the sauce ingredients in a blender and blend until smooth. Set aside.

2. Coat a large nonstick skillet with the oil and preheat over medium-high heat. Add the scallops and cook, stirring frequently for several minutes, until the scallops turn opaque and are cooked through.

3. Pour the sauce over the scallops and cook, stirring constantly for another minute or two, until the sauce is heated through and thickens slightly. Serve hot, topping each serving with a sprinkling of scallions and cilantro or parsley.

Nutritional Facts (per serving)
CALORIES: 239 CARBOHYDRATES: 13 g
CHOLESTEROL: 47 mg FAT: 8.6 g SAT. FAT: 0.9 g
FIBER: 0.7 g PROTEIN: 27 g SODIUM: 569 mg
CALCIUM: 46 mg
   Diabetic exchanges: 3 very lean meat, ½ fruit, 1½ fat

▪ ▪ ▪

Grecian-style Grouper

YIELD: 4 SERVINGS

4 grouper fillets (5 ounces each)
1 tablespoon Greek seasoning*
1 tablespoon plus 1 teaspoon extra virgin
   olive oil

TOPPING
4 cups chopped fresh spinach
2 medium plum tomatoes, diced

1 teaspoon crushed garlic

2 tablespoons dry white wine

¼ cup reduced-fat feta cheese (plain or with
   sun-dried tomatoes and herbs)

1. Rinse the fillets with cool water and pat dry with paper towels. Sprinkle both sides of each fish fillet with some of the Greek seasoning.

2. Coat a large nonstick skillet with the olive oil and preheat over medium-high heat. Add the fish and cook for several minutes, until nicely browned on the bottom. Turn the fillets, cover, and cook for several minutes more, until the fish turns opaque and flakes easily with a fork. Remove the fish from the skillet and set aside to keep warm.

3. Add the spinach, tomatoes, garlic, and wine to the skillet. Cook over medium-high heat for a couple of minutes, until the spinach is wilted and the tomatoes just begin to soften. Add a little more wine if the skillet starts to dry out, but only enough to prevent scorching.

4. Place a fish fillet on each of 4 serving plates and top each fillet with a quarter of the vegetable mixture and a sprinkling of the feta cheese. Serve hot.

Nutritional Facts (per serving)

CALORIES: 218 CARBOHYDRATES: 3 g
CHOLESTEROL: 57 mg FAT: 8.2 g SAT. FAT: 2.2 g
FIBER: 1 g PROTEIN: 32 g SODIUM: 482 mg
CALCIUM: 108 mg

   Diabetic exchanges: 3 very lean meat, 1 vegetable, 1 fat

*To make homemade, reduced-sodium Greek seasoning, combine 1 tablespoon each oregano, rosemary, lemon pepper, and onion powder with 2 teaspoons garlic powder and 1 teaspoon salt. Store leftovers in a jar for up to 6 months.

■ ■ ■

Salmon with Roasted Plum Tomatoes

YIELD: 4 SERVINGS

TOPPING

4 medium-large plum tomatoes, cut into ¾-inch
   chunks

1 tablespoon balsamic vinegar

1 teaspoon crushed garlic

¼ teaspoon dried oregano

4 boneless skinless salmon fillets (5 ounces
   each)

¼ teaspoon salt

½ teaspoon coarsely ground black pepper

olive oil cooking spray

¼ cup thinly sliced scallions

1. Preheat oven to 450°.

2. Combine the topping ingredients in a bowl and toss to mix well. Set aside.

3. Rinse the salmon fillets with cool water and pat dry with paper towels. Sprinkle both sides of each fillet with some of the salt and pepper. Coat a medium baking sheet with nonstick cooking spray and arrange the fillets

on the pan. Spray the tops lightly with the cooking spray. Coat another medium baking sheet with cooking spray and spread the tomato mixture over the sheet.

4. Place both baking sheets in the oven and bake for about 10 minutes, until the fish flakes easily with a fork and the tomatoes are tender but not mushy. If the tomatoes are done before the fish is, remove them from the oven and set aside to keep warm. Serve the fillets hot, topping each serving with some of the tomatoes and a sprinkling of scallions.

Nutritional Facts (per serving)

CALORIES: 219 CARBOHYDRATES: 4 g
CHOLESTEROL: 78 mg FAT: 9.2 g SAT. FAT: 1.4 g
FIBER: 0.8 g PROTEIN: 29 g SODIUM: 215 mg
CALCIUM: 26 mg

Diabetic exchanges: 3 lean meat, 1 vegetable

■ ■ ■

Citrus-glazed Fish Fillets

YIELD: 4 SERVINGS

4 orange roughy or cod fillets (5-ounces each)
¼ teaspoon ground black pepper
1 tablespoon canola oil
3 tablespoons thinly sliced scallions

GLAZE
¼ cup orange juice
2 tablespoons light (low-sugar) orange
  marmalade

2 tablespoons reduced-sodium soy sauce
1 teaspoon sesame oil
½ teaspoon ground ginger

1. Rinse the fillets and pat dry with paper towels. Sprinkle each fillet with some of the pepper. Coat a large nonstick skillet with the canola oil and preheat over medium-high heat. Add the fillets and cook for about 3 minutes on each side, until the fish is nicely browned and flakes easily with a fork. Remove from the skillet and set aside to keep warm.

2. Add all of the sauce ingredients to the skillet and cook over medium-high heat, stirring frequently for several minutes or until the sauce is reduced by half. Drizzle the sauce over the fish fillets and top with a sprinkling of scallions. Serve hot.

Nutritional Facts (per serving)

CALORIES: 157 CARBOHYDRATES: 5 g
CHOLESTEROL: 28 mg FAT: 5.6 g SAT. FAT: 0.4 g
FIBER: 0.2 g PROTEIN: 21 g SODIUM: 540 mg
CALCIUM: 47 mg

Diabetic exchanges: 3 very lean meat, ⅓ other carbohydrate, 1 fat

■ ■ ■

Crispy Oven-fried Fish

YIELD: 4 SERVINGS

SAUCE

¼ cup nonfat or light mayonnaise

1 tablespoon finely chopped capers

2 teaspoons finely chopped onion

4 cod, orange roughy, flounder, or other white
    fish fillets (5 ounces each)

¼ cup plus 2 tablespoons fat-free egg substitute

¼ cup plus 2 tablespoons finely ground
    Special-K cereal crumbs

¼ cup grated Parmesan cheese

½ teaspoon dried Italian seasoning

olive oil cooking spray

1. Preheat oven to 450°.

2. To make the sauce, combine all of the sauce ingredients in a small bowl and stir to mix well. Set aside.

3. Rinse the fish with cool water and pat it dry with paper towels. Set aside.

4. Place the egg substitute in a shallow dish. Place the cereal crumbs, Parmesan cheese, and Italian seasoning in another shallow dish and stir to mix well. Dip the fish pieces first in the egg substitute and then in the crumb mixture, turning to coat both sides well.

5. Coat a medium-sized baking sheet with the cooking spray and arrange the fish fillets on the sheet. Spray the tops lightly with the cooking spray and bake for 12 to 15 minutes, until the outside is crisp and golden and the fish flakes easily with a fork. Serve hot, accompanied by the sauce.

Nutritional Facts (per serving)

CALORIES: 194 CARBOHYDRATES: 9 g
CHOLESTEROL: 65 mg FAT: 3 g SAT. FAT: 1.2 g
FIBER: 0.4 g PROTEIN: 31 g SODIUM: 457 mg
CALCIUM: 106 mg

   Diabetic exchanges: 3 very lean meat, ½ starch

■ ■ ■

Grilled Scallop Kebabs

YIELD: 4 SERVINGS

1¼ pounds large scallops

8 pieces (1-inch each) red or yellow bell
    pepper

8 pieces (1-inch each) green bell pepper

8 frozen small whole onions, thawed

1 teaspoon fines herbes or Italian seasoning

¾ teaspoon lemon pepper

½ teaspoon garlic powder

¼ teaspoon salt

1 tablespoon plus 1 teaspoon extra virgin
    olive oil

1. Rinse the scallops and pat dry with paper towels. Place in a large bowl along with the peppers and onions. Add the fines herbes or Italian seasoning, lemon pepper, garlic powder, salt, and olive oil and toss to mix.

2. Thread a quarter of the scallops and vegetables onto four 14-inch skewers. (Leave a little space between the ingredients to ensure even cooking.)

3. Coat a grill rack with olive oil and grill covered over medium coals for several minutes on each side, until nicely browned and the shrimp or scallops are cooked through. Alternatively, cook for several minutes on each side under a preheated broiler. Serve hot.

Nutritional Facts (per serving)

CALORIES: 182 CARBOHYDRATES: 7 g
CHOLESTEROL: 47 mg FAT: 5.7 g SAT. FAT: 0.7 g
FIBER: 1 g PROTEIN: 24 g SODIUM: 475 mg
    Diabetic exchanges: 4 very lean meat, 1 vegetable, 1 fat

■ ■ ■

16. SATISFYING THE SWEET TOOTH

You may be happy to learn that living a diabetes prevention lifestyle does not have to mean giving up desserts. Having said that, moderation is still the best policy when it comes to sweets, so include them in your diet with your weight and personal nutrition goals in mind. Also, some desserts are definitely better choices than others. For instance, most desserts can be improved by replacing saturated fats with more healthful oils and by cutting back on sugar and white flour where possible. In addition, sweet treats that contain fruits, dairy products, nuts, and whole grains can actually provide a respectable amount of nutrition.

This chapter features a dazzling array of lighter desserts. Each of the following recipes is designed to keep calories, fat, and carbohydrates to a minimum—without sacrificing taste. For instance, many of the recipes in this chapter take advantage of the natural sweetness of fruit, so only a small amount of added sugar is needed. Cakes are topped with simple glazes or light frostings instead of thick sugary icings. And puddings, custards, and mousses are made with lower-fat dairy products and light whipped toppings. In addition, many of these recipes include sugar-free or reduced-sugar ingredients, which helps keep carbs to a minimum.

Light Carrot Cake

YIELD: 20 SERVINGS

1 cup unbleached flour

1 cup oat flour

1 ¼ cups sugar

½ cup sugar substitute

1 ½ teaspoons baking soda

¼ teaspoon salt

2 teaspoons ground cinnamon

¼ cup apple juice

¾ cup fat-free egg substitute or 3 eggs, lightly beaten

½ cup canola oil

3 cups (not packed) grated carrots (about 6 medium)

1 ½ teaspoons vanilla extract

½ cup chopped walnuts

FROSTING

1 block (8 ounces) nonfat or reduced-fat cream cheese, softened to room temperature

Sugar substitute equal to ½ cup sugar

¼ cup instant cheesecake or vanilla pudding mix (use regular, not sugar-free)

¼ cup nonfat or low-fat milk

2 cups nonfat or light whipped topping

1. Preheat oven to 350°.

2. Place the flours, sugar, sugar substitute, baking soda, salt, and cinnamon in a large bowl and stir to mix well. Add the apple juice, egg substitute or eggs, oil, carrots, and vanilla extract and stir to mix well. Fold in the nuts.

3. Coat a 9 × 13-inch pan with nonstick cooking spray and spread the batter evenly in the pan. Bake for about 30 minutes, until the top springs back when lightly touched and a wooden toothpick inserted in the center of the cake comes out clean. Remove the cake from the oven and cool to room temperature.

4. To make the frosting, place the cream cheese and sugar substitute in a medium-sized bowl and beat with an electric mixer until smooth. Slowly beat in the milk. Add the pudding mix and beat for 1 minute to mix well. Fold in the whipped topping.

5. Spread the frosting over the cake, cover, and refrigerate for at least 3 hours before cutting into squares and serving.

Nutritional Facts (per serving)

CALORIES: 192 CARBOHYDRATES: 27 g

CHOLESTEROL: 1 mg FAT: 7.8 g SAT. FAT: 0.5 g

FIBER: 1.5 g PROTEIN: 4.1 g SODIUM: 216 mg

CALCIUM: 50 mg

Diabetic exchanges: 2 carbohydrate, 1½ fat

■ ■ ■

Cherry Fudge Cake

YIELD: 20 SERVINGS

1 box (1 pound, 2.25 ounces) chocolate fudge
    cake mix
20-ounce can no-added-sugar or light
    (reduced-sugar) cherry pie filling
¼ cup plus 2 tablespoons fat-free egg substitute
    or 2 eggs, lightly beaten
½ cup chopped walnuts (optional)

FROSTING
1¼ cups light vanilla yogurt
1 package (4-serving size) sugar-free instant
    white or dark chocolate pudding mix
2 to 3 cups nonfat or light whipped topping
3 tablespoons chopped walnuts
3 tablespoons shaved dark chocolate

1. Preheat oven to 350°.

2. Place the cake mix, cherry pie filling, and egg substitute or eggs in a large bowl and stir with a wooden spoon to mix well. Fold in the walnuts if desired. Coat a 9 × 13-inch pan with nonstick cooking spray and spread the batter evenly in the pan.

3. Bake for about 28 minutes, just until the top springs back when lightly touched and a wooden toothpick inserted in the center of the cake comes out clean or coated with a few fudgy crumbs. Be careful not to over-bake. Let the cake cool to room temperature.

4. To make the frosting, place the yogurt and pudding mix in a medium-sized bowl and beat with an electric mixer until smooth. Add the whipped topping and beat just until the topping is mixed in. Spread the frosting over the cooled cake and sprinkle the walnuts and chocolate over the top. Cover the cake and re-frigerate for at least 8 hours or overnight before serving (the cake will become moister as it sits).

Nutritional Facts (per serving)
CALORIES: 160 CARBOHYDRATES: 30 g CHOLESTEROL: 0 mg
FAT: 3 g SAT. FAT: 0.9 g FIBER: 1.1 g PROTEIN: 2.7 g
SODIUM: 293 mg CALCIUM: 51 mg
Diabetic exchanges: 2 carbohydrate, ½ fat

■ ■ ■

Light Cherry Cheesecake

YIELD: 8 SERVINGS

¼ cup nonfat or low-fat milk
1 teaspoon plain unflavored gelatin
8-ounce block nonfat or light (Neufchâtel)
    cream cheese
½ cup light vanilla or lemon yogurt
Sugar substitute equal to ½ cup plus 2
    tablespoons of sugar
½ teaspoon vanilla extract
1 Graham Cracker Graham Pie Crust (p. 223)
1½ cups no-added-sugar or lite cherry-pie filling

1. Place the milk in a small pot, sprinkle the gelatin over the top, and let it sit for

1 minute to allow the gelatin to soften. Place the pot over low heat and stir for several minutes or until the gelatin is completely dissolved (do not let the milk boil). Set aside for about 10 minutes to cool slightly.

2. Place the cream cheese, yogurt, sugar substitute, and vanilla in a medium bowl and beat until smooth. Slowly pour in the milk mixture and beat until smooth. Spread the cheese filling evenly into the pie crust and chill for at least 2 hours. Spread the pie filling over the top and chill for an additional hour or until the filling is set.

Nutritional Facts (per serving)

CALORIES: 197 CARBOHYDRATES: 26 g
CHOLESTEROL: 20 mg FAT: 6.2 g SAT. FAT: 1 g
FIBER: 1.7 g PROTEIN: 8.6 g SODIUM: 295 mg
CALCIUM: 128 mg

Diabetic exchanges: 2 carbohydrate, 1 fat

■ ■ ■

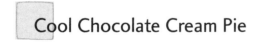

Cool Chocolate Cream Pie

YIELD: 8 SERVINGS

2 packages (4-serving size) sugar-free cook-and-serve chocolate pudding mix
pinch ground cinnamon (optional)
3½ cups nonfat or low-fat milk
1 Graham Cracker Pie Crust (on this page)
⅓ cup light vanilla yogurt
1½ cups nonfat or light whipped topping
2 tablespoons sliced almonds

1. Place pudding mix and cinnamon, if using, in a 2-quart glass bowl and slowly whisk in the milk. Microwave at high power for about 8 minutes, stirring every couple of minutes until the pudding is thickened and bubbly. Let the pudding cool for 5 minutes, stirring twice, and then pour the pudding into the crust. Place the pie in the refrigerator and chill uncovered for 2 hours.

2. Fold the yogurt into the whipped topping and spread over the pie, swirling the top. Sprinkle the almonds over the top. Cover and chill for an additional hour, until the filling is set, before serving.

Nutritional Facts (per serving)

CALORIES: 225 CARBOHYDRATES: 33 g
CHOLESTEROL: 2 mg FAT: 6.3 g SAT. FAT: 1.4 g
FIBER: 2.4 g PROTEIN: 8.5 g SODIUM: 287 mg
CALCIUM: 158 mg

Diabetic exchanges: 2 carbohydrate, 1 fat

■ ■ ■

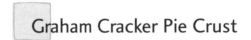

Graham Cracker Pie Crust

YIELD: 8 SERVINGS

¾ cup finely ground graham cracker crumbs
½ cup toasted wheat germ
2 tablespoons sugar
Sugar substitute equal to 3 tablespoons sugar
3 tablespoons melted margarine or butter
1 tablespoon fat-free egg substitute

1. Preheat oven to 350°.

2. Place the graham cracker crumbs, wheat germ, sugar, and sugar substitute in a food processor and process for about 15 seconds to mix well. Add the margarine or butter and the egg substitute and process, pulsing for a few seconds at a time, until the mixture is moist and crumbly and holds together when pinched. Add a little more egg substitute if the mixture seems too dry.

3. Coat a 9-inch pie pan with nonstick cooking spray and press the mixture firmly over the bottom and sides of the pan. Bake for about 8 minutes or until lightly browned. Let cool to room temperature before filling.

Nutritional Facts (per serving)
CALORIES: 127 CARBOHYDRATES: 16 g
CHOLESTEROL: 0 mg FAT: 6.2 g SAT. FAT: 1 g FIBER: 1.2 g
PROTEIN: 3 g SODIUM: 130 mg CALCIUM: 8 mg
  Diabetic exchanges: 1 carbohydrate, 1 fat

■ ■ ■

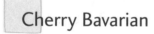

Cherry Bavarian

YIELD: 6 SERVINGS

2 cups frozen dark pitted sweet cherries,
  coarsely chopped and thawed
1 package (4-serving size) sugar-free cherry
  gelatin mix
1 ½ cups light vanilla yogurt
3 cups nonfat or light whipped topping

1. Drain the juice from the thawed cherries into a 1-cup glass measure and add enough water to bring the volume to ½ cup. Place the juice mixture in a microwave oven and heat at high power for a minute or two, until it comes to a boil.

2. Pour the boiling juice mixture into a large bowl. Sprinkle the gelatin over the top and stir with a wire whisk for 3 minutes, until the gelatin is completely dissolved. Set the mixture aside for about 15 minutes, until it reaches room temperature.

3. When the gelatin mixture has cooled to room temperature, whisk in the yogurt. Place the mixture in the refrigerator and chill for 15 minutes. Stir the mixture, it should be the consistency of pudding. If it is too thin, return it to the refrigerator for a few minutes.

4. When the gelatin mixture has reached the proper consistency, stir it with a wire whisk until smooth. Fold in first the cherries and then the whipped topping.

5. Divide the mixture among six 8-ounce wine glasses, cover, and chill for at least 3 hours before serving.

Nutritional Facts (per ¾-cup serving)
CALORIES: 143 CARBOHYDRATES: 27 g
CHOLESTEROL: 1 mg FAT: 1.2 g SAT. FAT: 0 g FIBER: 1.3 g
PROTEIN: 3.8 g SODIUM: 94 mg CALCIUM: 118 mg
  Diabetic exchanges: 2 carbohydrate

■ ■ ■

Chocolate-Peanut Butter Parfaits

YIELD: 4 SERVINGS

1 package (4-serving size) sugar-free
    instant or cook-and-serve chocolate
    pudding mix
2 cups nonfat or low-fat milk
2 tablespoons shaved dark chocolate
    (optional)

PEANUT BUTTER MIXTURE
3 tablespoons nonfat or low-fat milk
3 to 4 tablespoons smooth peanut butter
2 cups nonfat or light whipped topping

1. Prepare the pudding using the milk according to package directions. Chill well before assembling the parfaits.

2. To make the peanut butter mixture, combine the milk and peanut butter in a medium bowl and whisk until smooth. Fold in the whipped topping.

3. To assemble the parfaits, place ¼ cup of the pudding in the bottom of each of four 8-ounce balloon wine glasses. Top the pudding with ¼ cup of the peanut butter mixture. Top the peanut butter layer in each glass with a quarter of the remaining pudding and then a quarter of the remaining peanut butter mixture. Top each serving with a sprinkling of chocolate if desired. Cover and chill for at least 2 hours before serving.

Nutritional Facts (per serving)
CALORIES: 213 CARBOHYDRATES: 28 g CHOLESTEROL: 2 mg
FAT: 6.3 g SAT. FAT: 1.4 g FIBER: 0.9 g PROTEIN: 7.8 g
SODIUM: 225 mg CALCIUM: 169 mg
    Diabetic exchanges: 2 carbohydrate, 1 fat

■ ■ ■

Baked Pumpkin Custard

YIELD: 6 SERVINGS

1 cup canned or cooked mashed pumpkin
¾ cup plus 2 tablespoons fat-free egg substitute
¼ cup honey
¼ cup sugar
1 teaspoon vanilla extract
1 teaspoon ground cinnamon
½ teaspoon ground ginger
¼ teaspoon ground nutmeg
12-ounce can evaporated nonfat or low-fat milk

1. Preheat oven to 350°.

2. Combine all of the ingredients except for the evaporated milk in a medium bowl and whisk to mix well. Add the evaporated milk and whisk again.

3. Coat a 1½-quart round casserole dish with nonstick cooking spray and pour the mixture into the dish. Set the dish in a pan filled with enough hot water to come halfway up the sides of the dish.

4. Bake uncovered for about 1 hour 10 minutes, until a sharp knife inserted near the center of the dish comes out clean.

5. Let the pudding sit at room temperature for 1 hour. Serve slightly warm or cover and chill before serving. Top each serving with a dollop of whipped topping or a drizzle of honey and a sprinkling of toasted pecans if desired. Refrigerate leftovers.

Nutritional Facts (per ⅔ cup serving)
CALORIES: 148 CARBOHYDRATES: 29 g
CHOLESTEROL: 2 mg FAT: 0.1 g SAT. FAT: 0 g FIBER: 1.2 g
PROTEIN: 7.5 g SODIUM: 146 mg CALCIUM: 165 mg
   Diabetic exchanges: 2 carbohydrate

■ ■ ■

Banana Pudding Parfaits

YIELD: 4 SERVINGS

1 package (4-serving size) sugar-free cook-and-
   serve or instant vanilla or chocolate pudding mix
2 cups nonfat or low-fat milk
1½ cups sliced bananas (about 2 medium)
½ cup nonfat or light whipped topping
2 tablespoons shaved dark chocolate

1. Prepare the pudding with the milk according to package directions. (If using cook-and-serve pudding, let it chill before assembling the recipe.) Place 2 tablespoons of the pudding in the bottom of each of four 8-ounce balloon wine glasses.

2. Top the pudding in each glass with 3 tablespoons of the banana slices and 3 tablespoons of the pudding. Repeat the layers and then top each dessert with a quarter of the whipped topping and chocolate.

3. Cover and chill for at least 30 minutes before serving.

Nutritional Facts (per serving)
CALORIES: 153 CARBOHYDRATES: 30 g CHOLESTEROL: 2 mg
FAT: 2.4 g SAT. FAT: 1.1 g FIBER: 1.7 g PROTEIN: 5 g
SODIUM: 176 mg CALCIUM: 156 mg
   Diabetic exchanges: 2 carbohydrate

■ ■ ■

Golden Peanut Butter Cookies

YIELD: 40 COOKIES

1 cup whole-wheat pastry flour
¾ cup oat flour
Sugar substitute equal to ¼ cup sugar
¾ teaspoon baking soda
¾ teaspoon baking powder
⅔ cup peanut butter
¼ cup plus 2 tablespoons margarine or butter
¾ cup light brown sugar
¼ cup fat-free egg substitute
2 tablespoons pure maple syrup
1 teaspoon vanilla extract

1. Preheat oven to 350°.

2. Combine the flours, sugar substitute, baking soda, and baking powder in a bowl and stir to mix well. Set aside.

3. Combine the peanut butter, margarine, and brown sugar in a large bowl and beat with an electric mixer to mix well. Beat in the egg substitute, maple syrup, and vanilla extract. Add the flour mixture to the peanut butter mixture and beat to mix well.

4. Shape level tablespoonfuls of the dough into balls and arrange 1½ inches apart on un-greased baking sheets. Flatten each cookie to ¼-inch thickness by crisscrossing with the tines of a fork. Dip the tines of the fork lightly in sugar between each cookie if desired.

5. Bake for 10 to 12 minutes, until the bottoms of the cookies are golden brown. Remove the cookies and let sit for 2 minutes. Transfer the cookies to wire racks to cool completely.

Nutritional Facts (per cookie)

CALORIES: 77 CARBOHYDRATES: 9 g CHOLESTEROL: 0 mg FAT: 4 g SAT. FAT: 0.7 g FIBER: 0.9 g PROTEIN: 2 g SODIUM: 82 mg CALCIUM: 14 mg

   Diabetic exchanges: ½ carbohydrate, 1 fat

▪ ▪ ▪

Chocolate Chip-Raisin Cookies

For variety, substitute white chocolate chips for the semi-sweet chips and dried cranberries or cherries for the raisins.

YIELD: 50 COOKIES

½ **cup margarine or butter, softened to room temperature**

¾ **cup light brown sugar**

¼ **cup fat-free egg substitute or 2 egg whites**

1 **teaspoon vanilla extract**

⅔ **cup whole-wheat pastry flour**

⅔ **cup oat flour**

½ **teaspoon baking soda**

½ **teaspoon baking powder**

⅔ **cup semi-sweet chocolate chips**

⅔ **cup dark raisins**

1 ½ **cups chopped walnuts**

1. Preheat oven to 350°.

2. Place the margarine or butter in a large bowl. Add the sugar, and beat until smooth. Add the egg substitute or egg and the vanilla extract and beat until smooth.

3. Combine the flours, baking soda, and baking powder and stir to mix well. Add to the margarine mixture and beat to mix well. Stir in the chocolate chips, raisins, and nuts.

4. Drop rounded teaspoons of dough onto ungreased baking sheets. Flatten each cookie with the tip of a spoon to spread it out slightly. Bake for about 10 minutes, until golden brown. Let the cookies cool on the pan for 2 minutes then transfer to wire racks to cool completely. Store in an airtight container.

Nutritional Facts (per cookie)

CALORIES: 78 CARBOHYDRATES: 9 g CHOLESTEROL: 0 mg FAT: 4.7 g SAT. FAT: 0.8 g FIBER: 0.8 g PROTEIN: 1.6 g SODIUM: 46 mg CALCIUM: 11 mg

   Diabetic exchanges: ½ carbohydrate, 1 fat

▪ ▪ ▪

Melon with Fresh Berry Sauce

YIELD: 6 SERVINGS

3⅓ cups fresh or frozen (thawed and undrained)
　raspberries or blackberries
1½ tablespoons orange juice
½ teaspoon lemon juice
Sugar substitute equal to 3 tablespoons sugar
½ cantaloupe melon
½ honeydew melon

1.　Place 2 cups of the berries and all of the orange juice and lemon juice in a blender or food processor and process until smooth. Pour the mixture into a wire strainer and use the back of a spoon to push the mixture through the strainer and into a bowl. Discard the seeds. Stir the sugar substitute into the berry purée and set the sauce aside.

2.　Remove the seeds and rind from the melons. Cut each melon piece into 3 long wedges and then cut each wedge in half cross-wise to make a total of 12 shorter wedges. Using a sharp knife, slice each melon wedge lengthwise toward the point without cutting completely to the end and open each wedge into a fan shape.

3.　Place 2 tablespoons of the sauce on each of 6 dessert plates. Top the sauce on each plate with a cantaloupe and honeydew fan and garnish with some of the remaining fresh berries. Serve immediately.

Nutritional Facts (per serving)
CALORIES: 85　CARBOHYDRATES: 21 g
CHOLESTEROL: 0 mg　FAT: 0.2 g　SAT. FAT: 0 g　FIBER: 3.3 g
PROTEIN: 1.6 g　SODIUM: 41 mg　CALCIUM: 17 mg
　Diabetic exchanges: 1½ carbohydrate

■　■　■

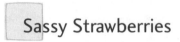

Sassy Strawberries

YIELD: 4 SERVINGS

3 cups sliced strawberries
3 tablespoons orange or raspberry liqueur
1½ tablespoons sugar
1½ tablespoons sugar substitute
Fresh mint leaves (optional)

1.　Place all of the ingredients except for the mint in a shallow bowl and toss to mix well.

2.　Cover and chill for 1 to 3 hours before serving. Garnish each serving with a couple of mint leaves if desired.

Nutritional Facts (per serving)
CALORIES: 99　CARBOHYDRATES: 19 g
CHOLESTEROL: 0 mg　FAT: 0.5 g　SAT. FAT: 0 g　FIBER: 2.9 g
PROTEIN: 0.8 g　SODIUM: 2 mg　CALCIUM: 18 mg
　Diabetic exchanges: 1¼ carbohydrate

■　■　■

Cinnamon-Peach Crisp

YIELD: 8 SERVINGS

2 cans (15 ounces each) sliced peaches in juice
2½ teaspoons cornstarch
Sugar substitute equal to ¼ cup sugar
¼ cup raisins (optional)

TOPPING

½ cup old-fashioned (5-minute) oats
3 tablespoons toasted wheat germ
¼ cup plus 2 tablespoons light brown sugar
1 teaspoon ground cinnamon
2 tablespoons soft reduced-fat margarine
½ cup chopped almonds or pecans

1. Preheat oven to 375°.
2. Drain the peaches, reserving ½ cup of the juice. Place the cornstarch in a 2-quart pot, add a tablespoon of the reserved juice, and stir to dissolve the cornstarch. Stir in the remaining reserved juice. Bring the mixture to a boil over medium-high heat. Cook and stir for a minute or two, until the juice has thickened. Stir in the sugar substitute, peaches, and if desired, the raisins and heat through.
3. Coat a 9-inch pie pan with cooking spray and spread the peach mixture evenly in the dish.
4. To make the topping, place the oats, wheat germ, brown sugar, and cinnamon in a medium bowl and stir to mix well. Add the margarine and stir until the mixture is moist and crumbly. Add a little more margarine if the mixture seems too dry. Stir in the nuts.

5. Sprinkle the topping over the fruit and bake uncovered for about 20 minutes, until the filling is bubbly around the edges and the topping is golden brown. Let sit for 20 minutes before serving.

Nutritional Facts (per serving)
CALORIES: 162 CARBOHYDRATES: 28 g
CHOLESTEROL: 0 mg FAT: 6 g SAT. FAT: 0.8 g FIBER: 2.7 g
PROTEIN: 3.8 g SODIUM: 32 mg CALCIUM: 37 mg
Diabetic exchanges: 2 carbohydrate, 1 fat

▪ ▪ ▪

Baked Pears with Citrus Sauce

YIELD: 6 SERVINGS

4½ medium firm but ripe pears, peeled, cored, and quartered lengthwise
¾ cup orange juice
¼ cup honey
¼ cup chopped toasted pecans (p. 233)

1. Preheat oven to 425°.
2. Coat a 9 × 13-inch pan with nonstick cooking spray and arrange the pears in a single layer in the pan. Combine the orange juice and honey in a small bowl and stir to mix well. Pour the orange juice mixture over the pears.

3. Bake uncovered for about 25 minutes, basting occasionally with the pan juices, until the pears are tender and the liquid is slightly syrupy.

4. Remove the dish from the oven and let sit for 10 minutes. Serve the pears warm drizzled with some of the juices. Top each serving with a sprinkling of the pecans.

Nutritional Facts (per serving)
CALORIES: 156 CARBOHYDRATES: 32 g
CHOLESTEROL: 0 mg FAT: 4.1 g SAT. FAT: 0.3 g
FIBER: 3.2 g PROTEIN: 1.2 g SODIUM: 1 mg
CALCIUM: 20 mg
    Diabetic exchanges: 2 carbohydrate, 1 fat

■ ■ ■

Sensational Berry Sundaes

YIELD: 4 SERVINGS

2 cups low-fat vanilla ice cream
1⅓ cups sliced strawberries or whole fresh
    raspberries
¼ cup lite (reduced-sugar) chocolate syrup
¼ cup sliced almonds

1. Place a ½-cup scoop of ice cream in each of 4 dessert dishes. Top the ice cream in each dish with a quarter of the berries.

2. Drizzle a tablespoon of the chocolate syrup over each dessert and top with a tablespoon of almonds. Serve immediately.

Nutritional Facts (per serving)
CALORIES: 179 CARBOHYDRATES: 29 g
CHOLESTEROL: 5 mg FAT: 5.5 g SAT. FAT: 1.3 g
FIBER: 2.9 g PROTEIN: 5.3 g SODIUM: 70 mg
CALCIUM: 122 mg
    Diabetic exchanges: 2 carbohydrate, 1 fat

■ ■ ■

Very Blueberry Sundaes

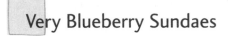

For variety, substitute coarsely chopped frozen cherries for the blueberries.

YIELD: 4 SERVINGS

SAUCE
1 cup frozen blueberries
3 tablespoons orange juice or 2 tablespoons
    orange juice plus 1 tablespoon orange liqueur
Sugar substitute equal to 2 tablespoons sugar

2 cups low-fat vanilla ice cream
¼ cup chopped toasted pecans or sliced toasted
    almonds (p. 233)

1. To make the sauce, place the blueberries, orange juice, and sugar substitute in a mini food processor and process until smooth. Set aside for about 15 minutes, until the mixture has thawed. Or transfer to a covered container and chill until ready to use.

2. To assemble the sundaes, place a ½-cup scoop of ice cream in each of 4 dessert dishes. Top the ice cream in each dish with a quarter

of the sauce and a sprinkling of the nuts. Serve immediately.

Nutritional Facts (per serving)
CALORIES: 176 CARBOHYDRATES: 25 g
CHOLESTEROL: 5 mg FAT: 7.6 g SAT. FAT: 1.5 g
FIBER: 2.8 g PROTEIN: 3.9 g SODIUM: 50 mg
CALCIUM: 110 mg
    Diabetic exchanges: 1½ carbohydrate, 1½ fat

■ ■ ■

Apple-Pecan Ice Cream Sundaes

YIELD: 4 SERVINGS

1 cup chopped no-added-sugar or reduced-sugar apple pie filling
2 cups low-fat vanilla ice cream
¼ cup chopped toasted pecans (p. 233)
ground cinnamon

1. Place the pie filling in a microwave-safe bowl and microwave at 60% power for about a minute to warm through.

2. Place a ½-cup scoop of ice cream in each of 4 dessert dishes. Top the ice cream in each dish with a quarter of the pie filling and a sprinkling of the nuts and cinnamon. Serve immediately.

Nutritional Facts (per serving)
CALORIES: 170 CARBOHYDRATES: 24 g
CHOLESTEROL: 5 mg FAT: 7.3 g SAT. FAT: 1.5 g
FIBER: 2.5 g PROTEIN: 3.7 g SODIUM: 57 mg
CALCIUM: 105 mg
    Diabetic exchanges: 1½ carbohydrate, 1½ fat

■ ■ ■

THE PROS AND CONS OF "SUGAR-FREE" ICE CREAM

Countless brands of sugar-free ice cream are available these days, but do be aware that some of these products contain just as many calories as the regular versions. Sugar-free ice cream is typically sweetened with a combination of sugar alcohols and artificial sweeteners.

Sugar alcohols contain about half the calories of regular sugar and are more slowly absorbed, which can offer an advantage. However, eating too much sugar alcohol can cause gas and bloating and have a laxative effect. In addition, to make up for the textural properties that are lost when sugar is left out, some sugar-free ice creams contain extra fat, offsetting any calorie savings gained from reducing sugar. So read labels carefully and be sure to consider calories before you buy.

Pear & Walnut Bread

YIELD: 16 SLICES

1-pound can sliced pears in juice

1 cup whole-wheat pastry flour

1 cup oat flour

⅓ cup sugar

Sugar substitute equal to ½ cup sugar

2 teaspoons baking powder

¼ teaspoon baking soda

¼ teaspoon ground cardamom or nutmeg

⅛ teaspoon salt

¼ cup canola oil

¼ cup fat-free egg substitute or 1 egg, beaten

1 teaspoon vanilla extract

¾ cup chopped walnuts or toasted pecans
   (p. 233)

1. Preheat over to 350°.

2. Drain the pears, reserving the juice, and place in a blender. Process the pears until smooth and pour into a 2-cup measure. Add enough of the reserved juice to bring the volume to 1 cup plus 2 tablespoons. Set aside.

3. Place the flours, sugar, sugar substitute, baking powder, baking soda, cardamom or nutmeg, and salt in a medium bowl and stir to mix well. Add the blended pears, oil, egg substitute or egg, and vanilla extract and stir to mix well. Stir in the nuts.

4. Coat an 8 × 4-inch pan with cooking spray. Spread the batter evenly in the pan and bake for about 40 minutes, until a wooden toothpick inserted in the center of the loaf comes out clean.

5. Let the bread cool in the pan for 15 minutes, then remove from the pan and place on a wire rack to cool completely.

Nutritional Facts (per slice)

CALORIES: 143 CARBOHYDRATES: 17 g CHOLESTEROL: 0 mg FAT: 7.2 g SAT. FAT: 0.5 g FIBER: 2.5 g PROTEIN: 3.8 g SODIUM: 108 mg CALCIUM: 46 mg

Diabetic exchanges: 1 carbohydrate, 1½ fat

▪ ▪ ▪

Apricot-Pecan Bread

YIELD: 16 SLICES

1-pound can apricots in juice

1 cup whole-wheat pastry flour

1 cup oat flour

⅓ cup sugar

Sugar substitute equal to ½ cup sugar

2 teaspoons baking powder

¼ teaspoon baking soda

⅛ teaspoon salt

¼ cup canola oil

¼ cup fat-free egg substitute or 1 egg, beaten

1 teaspoon vanilla extract

⅓ cup finely chopped dried apricots

½ cup chopped toasted pecans (p. 233)

1. Preheat oven to 350°.

2. Drain the apricots, reserving the juice,

and place in a blender. Process the apricots until smooth and pour into a 2-cup measure. Add enough of the reserved juice to bring the volume to 1 cup plus 2 tablespoons. Set aside.

3. Place the flours, sugar, sugar substitute, baking powder, baking soda, and salt in a medium bowl and stir to mix well. Add the blended apricots, oil, egg substitute or egg, and vanilla extract and stir to mix well. Stir in the dried apricots and pecans.

4. Coat an 8 × 4-inch pan with cooking spray. Spread the batter evenly in the pan and bake for about 40 minutes, until a wooden toothpick inserted in the center of the loaf comes out clean.

5. Let the bread cool in the pan for 15 minutes, then remove from the pan and place on a wire rack to cool completely.

Nutritional Facts (per slice)

CALORIES: 134 CARBOHYDRATES: 17 g
CHOLESTEROL: 0 mg FAT: 6.6 g SAT. FAT: 0.5 g
FIBER: 2.5 g PROTEIN: 2.9 g SODIUM: 77 mg
CALCIUM: 10 mg
    Diabetic exchanges: 1 carbohydrate, 1 fat

■ ■ ■

TOASTING NUTS

To bring out the flavor of nuts, try toasting them. Toasting nuts intensifies their flavors and can transform a dish from ordinary into extraordinary. To toast nuts, simply arrange the desired amount in a single layer on a baking sheet and bake at 350 degrees until lightly browned with a toasted, nutty aroma. Chopped or sliced nuts will be done in as little as five minutes, while whole or halved nuts will take a few minutes longer. Just be careful to watch them closely during the last part of baking as they can become burned very quickly. To save time, toast a little extra and store leftovers in the freezer or refrigerator.

Appendix A: Body Mass Index Table

BODY MASS INDEX TABLE										
HEALTHY WEIGHT						**OVERWEIGHT**				
BMI	**19**	**20**	**21**	**22**	**23**	**24**	**25**	**26**	**27**	**28**	**29**
Height	*Body Weight (pounds)*										
4'10"	91	96	100	105	110	115	119	124	129	134	138
4'11"	94	99	104	109	114	119	124	128	133	138	143
5'0"	97	102	107	112	118	123	128	133	138	143	148
5'1"	100	106	111	116	122	127	132	137	143	148	153
5'2"	104	109	115	120	126	131	136	142	147	153	158
5'3"	107	113	118	124	130	135	141	146	152	158	163
5'4"	110	116	122	128	134	140	145	151	157	163	169
5'5"	114	120	126	132	138	144	150	156	162	168	174
5'6"	118	124	130	136	142	148	155	161	167	173	179
5'7"	121	127	134	140	146	153	159	166	172	178	185
5'8"	125	131	138	144	151	158	164	171	177	184	190
5'9"	128	135	142	149	155	162	169	176	182	189	196
5'10"	132	139	146	153	160	167	174	181	188	195	202
5'11"	136	143	150	157	165	172	179	186	193	200	208
6'0"	140	147	154	162	169	177	184	191	199	206	213
6'1"	144	151	159	166	174	182	189	197	204	212	219
6'2"	148	155	163	171	179	186	194	202	210	218	225
6'3"	152	160	168	176	184	192	200	208	216	224	232
6'4"	156	164	172	180	189	197	205	213	221	230	238

Adapted from *The Practical Guide to the Indentification, Evaluation, and Treatment of Overweight and Obesity in Adults.* National Institutes of Health; National Heart, Lung, and Blood Institute; North American Association for the Study of Obesity. NIH Publication number 00-4084, October 2000. (Accessed 11/20/03 at http://www.nhlbi.nih.gov/guidelines/obesity/prctgd_b.pdf).

BODY MASS INDEX TABLE

OBESE

30	31	32	33	34	35	36	37	38	39	40
Body Weight (pounds)										
143	148	153	158	162	167	172	177	181	186	191
148	153	158	163	168	173	178	183	188	193	198
153	158	163	168	174	179	184	189	194	199	204
158	164	169	174	180	185	190	195	201	206	211
164	169	175	180	186	191	196	202	207	213	218
169	175	180	186	191	197	203	208	214	220	225
174	180	186	192	197	204	209	215	221	227	232
180	186	192	198	204	210	216	222	228	234	240
186	192	198	204	210	216	223	229	235	241	247
191	198	204	211	217	223	230	236	242	249	255
197	203	210	216	223	230	236	243	249	256	262
203	209	216	223	230	236	243	250	257	263	270
209	216	222	229	236	243	250	257	264	271	278
215	222	229	236	243	250	257	265	272	279	286
221	228	235	242	250	258	265	272	279	287	294
227	235	242	250	257	265	272	280	288	295	302
233	241	249	256	264	272	280	287	295	303	311
240	248	256	264	272	279	287	295	303	311	319
246	254	263	271	279	287	295	304	312	320	328

Appendix B: Sample Menus

This section helps you put things in perspective by offering fourteen days of diabetes-prevention meal plans. The following menus present a series of options ranging from 1,200 to 2,100 calories per day. The intent of this section is not to have you adhere to a strictly regimented eating plan, but rather to demonstrate some meal-planning possibilities. The following menus are moderate in carbohydrate and emphasize "good" carbs such as vegetables, fruits, and whole grains to help keep blood sugar and insulin levels under control. Additional emphasis is placed on unsaturated fats, lean proteins, and low-fat dairy products to foster excellent health for many years to come.

How Many Calories Do You Need?

Calorie needs vary greatly depending on your activity level, genetics, and gender. However, most people need about 13 to 15 calories per pound to maintain their body weight. So you can estimate your calorie needs by multiplying your goal weight by 13 to 15. For instance, if your goal weight is 140 pounds, you will probably need somewhere between 1,820 and 2,100 calories per day to maintain that weight. If you start consuming that amount of calories, you should gradually reach your goal and maintain at that level. To reach your goal faster, you can cut back a bit more, increase your activity level, or do some combination of the two.

One word of warning: Cutting back is crucial for anyone who wants to reduce their weight, but don't get overzealous and cut back too much. In general, women should not eat less than 1,200 calories per day and men should not eat less than 1,500 calories. By going below these levels, you risk slowing your metabolism.

How to Simplify

The following menus feature recipes from this book, but you can also improvise with convenience and restaurant foods. For instance, instead of making soup from scratch, choose a similar canned variety, choosing a brand made with less salt and fat. Instead of making a main dish salad from scratch, substitute a similar fast food salad. Just be sure to go easy on the dressing and limit toppings like fried rice noodles, croutons, and other refined carbs. Instead of a homemade turkey wrap, substitute a turkey sandwich on whole-wheat bread. No time to cook an omelette? Scramble some egg substitute in the microwave or have a couple of ounces of another lean protein like turkey instead.

Adapting Menus to Suit Your Taste

You can also adapt the following menus to suit your individual preferences. For instance, instead of low-fat cole slaw, substitute another low-carb vegetable like a garden salad or a serving of green beans or broccoli. Instead of chicken, have lean beef, pork, or fish. It's important to customize meals to suit your personal tastes. Realize though, if you substitute similar foods with higher-calorie ingredients, your daily calorie intake will rise accordingly.

Meal & Snack Patterns

The following menus feature 3 meals plus 1 mid-afternoon snack, but you can adapt this somewhat to suit your preferences. For instance, if you also want a mid-morning snack, you can save something from breakfast, such as a piece of fruit or a hard-boiled egg, and have it a little later.

Daily Calorie Level	1,200	1,500	1,800	2,100
BREAKFAST	Ham, Egg, & Cheese Breakfast Pitas (p. 122) Cup of mixed fresh berries	Ham, Egg, & Cheese Breakfast Pitas (p. 122) Cup of mixed fresh berries 1 cup nonfat or low-fat milk	Ham, Egg, & Cheese Breakfast Pitas (p. 122) Cup of mixed fresh berries 1 cup nonfat or low-fat milk	Ham, Egg, & Cheese Breakfast Pitas (p. 122) Cup of mixed fresh berries 1 cup nonfat or low-fat milk
LUNCH	West Coast Cobb Salad (p. 153)	West Coast Cobb Salad (p. 153)	West Coast Cobb Salad (p. 153) 1 cup Lentil Soup with Spinach & Potatoes (p. 149)	West Coast Cobb Salad (p. 153) 1 cup Lentil Soup with Spinach & Potatoes (p. 149)
SNACK	8 oz. light yogurt	8 oz. light yogurt 2 TBSP honey crunch wheat germ ½ cup blueberries	8 oz. light yogurt 2 TBSP honey crunch wheat germ ½ cup blueberries	8 oz. light yogurt 3 TBSP walnuts ½ cup blueberries
DINNER	Slow-cooked Sicilian Pot Roast (p. 211) with ½ cup whole-wheat pasta ⅔ cup Garlicky Green Beans (p. 170)	Slow-cooked Sicilian Pot Roast (p. 211) with ½ cup whole-wheat pasta ⅔ cup Garlicky Green Beans (p. 170)	1½ servings Slow-cooked Sicilian Pot Roast (p. 211) with ½ cup whole-wheat pasta ⅔ cup Garlicky Green Beans (p. 170)	1½ servings Slow-cooked Sicilian Pot Roast (p. 211) with 1 cup whole-wheat pasta ⅔ cup Garlicky Green Beans (p. 170)

DINNER *(continued)*	Orange-Onion Salad (p. 162)	Orange-Onion Salad (p. 162)	Orange-Onion Salad (p. 162)	Orange-Onion Salad (p. 162) 1 piece Light Cherry Cheesecake (p. 222)
TOTAL CALORIES:	1,267	1,446	1,723	2,096
CARBS (G):	128	159	190	229
FAT (G):	39	41	47	66
SAT. FAT (G):	6.7	7.2	9.1	11
CHOL. (MG):	272	277	319	339
PROTEIN (G):	105	118	142	156
FIBER (G):	29	31	39	45
SODIUM (MG):	2,246	2,380	3,092	3,388
CALCIUM (MG):	934	1,247	1,360	1,506
% CARB	40	43	43	43
% PROTEIN	33	32	33	29
% FAT	27	25	24	28

Daily Calorie Level	1,200	1,500	1,800	2,100
BREAKFAST	Berry Breakfast Parfait (p. 124)	Berry Breakfast Parfait (p. 124) 1 hard-boiled egg	Berry Breakfast Parfait (p. 124) 1 hard-boiled egg	Berry Breakfast Parfait (p. 124) 1 hard-boiled egg
LUNCH	Colossal Club Wraps (p. 182) 1 stalk celery filled with 1 TBSP natural peanut butter	Colossal Club Wraps (p. 182) 1 cup Garden Garbanzo Soup (p. 148) 1 stalk celery filled with 1½ TBSP natural peanut butter	Colossal Club Wraps (p. 182) 1 cup Garden Garbanzo Soup (p. 148) 1 stalk celery filled with 2 TBSP natural peanut butter	Colossal Club Wraps (p. 182) 1 cup Garden Garbanzo Soup (p. 148) 1 stalk celery filled with 2 TBSP natural peanut butter
SNACK	Medium apple 1½ ounces low-fat cheese	Large apple 1½ ounces low-fat cheese	Large apple 1½ ounces low-fat cheese	Large apple 2 ounces low-fat cheese
DINNER	Pork Chops with Mushrooms & Onions (p. 213) 1 serving Simply Baked Spaghetti Squash (p. 177) 1 cup Easy Oven-baked Vegetables (p. 170)	Pork Chops with Mushrooms & Onions (p. 213) 1 serving Simply Baked Spaghetti Squash (p. 177) 1 cup Easy Oven-baked Vegetables (p. 170)	Pork Chops with Mushrooms & Onions (p. 213) 1 serving Simply Baked Spaghetti Squash (p. 177) 1 cup Easy Oven-baked Vegetables (p. 170) 1 slice Cool Chocolate Cream Pie (p. 223)	2 servings Pork Chops with Mushrooms & Onions (p. 213) 2 servings Simply Baked Spaghetti Squash (p. 177) 1 cup Easy Oven-baked Vegetables (p. 170) 1 slice Cool Chocolate Cream Pie (p. 223)

TOTAL CALORIES:	1,170	1,481	1,753	2,006
CARBS (G):	125	160	194	207
FAT (G):	35	48	58	69
SAT. FAT (G):	8.8	10.9	12.9	15.6
CHOL. (MG):	145	335	337	395
PROTEIN (G):	89	104	114	138
FIBER (G):	20	28	31	34
SODIUM (MG):	1,999	2,534	2,841	3,174
CALCIUM (MG):	1,155	1,232	1,394	1,444
% CARB	43	43	44	42
% PROTEIN	30	28	26	27
% FAT	27	29	30	31

Daily Calorie Level	1,200	1,500	1,800	2,100
BREAKFAST	½ cup scrambled egg substitute	½ cup scrambled egg substitute	½ cup scrambled egg substitute	½ cup scrambled egg substitute
	½ cup Creamy Cheese Grits (p. 126)	½ cup Creamy Cheese Grits (p. 126)	¾ cup Creamy Cheese Grits (p. 126)	¾ cup Creamy Cheese Grits (p. 126)
	1 cup diced honey-dew melon	1 cup diced honey-dew melon	1 cup diced honey-dew melon	1 cup diced honey-dew melon
	Vegetarian sausage patty	Vegetarian sausage patty	Vegetarian sausage patty	Vegetarian sausage patty
LUNCH	1 cup Savory Chili (p.145) with 2 TBSP low-fat cheese	1½ cups Savory Chili (p. 145) with 2 TBSP low-fat cheese	2 cups Savory Chili (p. 145) with 3 TBSP low-fat cheese	2 cups Savory Chili (p. 145) with 3 TBSP low-fat cheese
	Fresh raw veggies with 2 TBSP light ranch dressing	Fresh raw veggies with 2 TBSP light ranch dressing	Fresh raw veggies with 3 TBSP light ranch dressing	Fresh raw veggies with 3 TBSP light ranch dressing
SNACK	8 ounces light yogurt	Frosty Fruit Smoothie (p. 125)	Frosty Fruit Smoothie (p. 125)	Frosty Fruit Smoothie (p. 125)
	1 TBSP walnuts	2 TBSP walnuts	¼ cup walnuts	¼ cup walnuts
DINNER	Scallops with Peanut Sauce (p. 215)	Scallops with Peanut Sauce (p. 215)	Scallops with Peanut Sauce (p. 215)	Scallops with Peanut Sauce (p. 215)
	Broiled Asparagus (p. 169)	Broiled Asparagus (p. 169)	Broiled Asparagus (p. 169)	Broiled Asparagus (p. 169)
	½ cup Colorful Rice pilaf (p. 175)	½ cup Colorful Rice pilaf (p. 175)	½ cup Colorful Rice pilaf (p. 175)	½ cup Colorful Rice pilaf (p. 175)
				1 oz. dark chocolate

TOTAL CALORIES:	1222	1491	1792	2048
CARBS (G):	132	170	197	228
FAT (G):	33	40	55	69
SAT. FAT (G):	6.1	7.3	9.3	16.6
CHOL. (MG):	105	122	145	149
PROTEIN (G):	99	116	133	139
FIBER (G):	23	34	41	44
SODIUM (MG):	2528	2792	3266	3425
CALCIUM (MG):	843	1234	1340	1432
% CARB	43	45	44	44
% PROTEIN	32	31	29	28
% FAT	25	24	27	31

Daily Calorie Level	1,200	1,500	1,800	2,100
BREAKFAST	Ham & Asparagus Omelette (p. 117) 1 cup sliced strawberries & diced mango	Ham & Asparagus Omelette (p. 117) 1 cup sliced strawberries & diced mango 1 slice whole-grain toast with 1 tsp trans-free margarine	Ham & Asparagus Omelette (p. 117) 1 cup sliced strawberries & diced mango 1 slice whole-grain toast with 1 tsp trans-free margarine	Ham & Asparagus Omelet (p. 117) 1 cup sliced strawberries & diced mango 1 slice whole-grain toast with 1 tsp trans-free margarine
LUNCH	Mediterranean Tuna Melts (p. 182) 6 baby carrots	Mediterranean Tuna Melts (p. 182) 6 baby carrots 1 cup Cream of Asparagus Soup (p. 145)	Mediterranean Tuna Melts (p. 182) Fresh raw veggies with 2 TBSP light ranch dressing 1 cup Cream of Asparagus Soup (p. 145)	Mediterranean Tuna Melts (p. 182) Fresh raw veggies with 2 TBSP light ranch dressing 1 cup Cream of Asparagus Soup (p. 145)
SNACK	1 cup nonfat or low-fat milk 3 TBSP almonds	1 cup nonfat or low-fat milk ¼ cup almonds	1 cup nonfat or low-fat milk ⅓ cup almonds	1 cup nonfat or low-fat milk ⅓ cup almonds
DINNER	Garden Meatloaf (p. 209) ¾ cup Dilled New Potatoes & Peas (p. 175) ⅔ cup Summer Squash with Onions & Herbs (p. 178)	Garden Meatloaf (p. 209) ¾ cup Dilled New Potatoes & Peas (p. 175) ⅔ cup Summer Squash with Onions & Herbs (p. 178)	1½ pieces Garden Meatloaf (p. 209) 1 cup Dilled New Potatoes & Peas (p. 175) 1 cup Summer Squash with Onions & Herbs (p. 178)	2 pieces Garden Meatloaf (p. 209) 1 cup Dilled New Potatoes & Peas (p. 175) 1 cup Summer Squash with Onions & Herbs (p. 178)

DINNER (continued)				1 oz dark chocolate
TOTAL CALORIES:	1,207	1,467	1,808	2,057
CARBS (G):	134	163	190	211
FAT (G):	31	44	62	76
SAT. FAT (G):	6.8	8.7	11	18.5
CHOL. (MG):	115	117	155	185
PROTEIN (G):	100	112	131	146
FIBER (G):	24	29	36	38
SODIUM (MG):	2,461	3,057	3,687	3,891
CALCIUM (MG):	967	1,138	1,199	1,229
% CARB	44	43	41	40
% PROTEIN	33	30	28	28
% FAT	23	27	30	32

Daily Calorie Level	1,200	1,500	1,800	2,100
BREAKFAST	Double Bran Muffins (p. 127) 1 cup nonfat or low-fat milk 1 medium orange	Double Bran Muffins (p. 127) 1 cup nonfat or low-fat milk 1 medium orange 1 hard-boiled egg	Double Bran Muffins (p. 127) 1 cup nonfat or low-fat milk 1 medium orange 1 hard-boiled egg	2 Double Bran Muffins (p. 127) 1 cup nonfat or low-fat milk 1 medium orange 1 hard-boiled egg
LUNCH	Southwestern Chicken Caesar Salad (p. 153) 2 TBSP chocolate-covered almonds	Southwestern Chicken Caesar Salad (p. 153) 1 cup Black Bean & Sausage Soup (p. 149) 3 TBSP chocolate-covered almonds	Southwestern Chicken Caesar Salad (p. 153) 1 cup Black Bean & Sausage Soup (p. 149) ¼ cup chocolate-covered almonds	Southwestern Chicken Caesar Salad (p. 153) 1 cup Black Bean & Sausage Soup (p. 149) ⅓ cup chocolate-covered almonds
SNACK	¼ cup low-fat tuna salad with 2 celery stalks	¼ cup low-fat tuna salad with 2 celery stalks	⅓ cup low-fat tuna salad with 2 celery stalks	½ cup low-fat tuna salad with 3 celery stalks
DINNER	Slimmed-Down Sloppy Joe on a light wheat bun (p. 188) ⅔ cup Crunchy Cabbage Salad (p. 166) ¼ medium cantaloupe	Slimmed-Down Sloppy Joe a light wheat bun (p. 188) ⅔ cup Crunchy Cabbage Salad (p. 166) ¼ medium cantaloupe	2 Slimmed-Down Sloppy Joes on light wheat buns (p. 188) ⅔ cup Crunchy Cabbage Salad (p. 166) ¼ medium cantaloupe	2 Slimmed-Down Sloppy Joes on light wheat buns (p. 188) 1 cup Crunchy Cabbage Salad (p. 166) ¼ medium cantaloupe

TOTAL CALORIES:	1,212	1,523	1,831	2,057
CARBS (G):	135	165	200	226
FAT (G):	42	53	62	71
SAT. FAT (G):	10.8	13	15.2	16.6
CHOL. (MG):	144	348	392	405
PROTEIN (G):	85	106	130	146
FIBER (G):	23	32	39	44
SODIUM (MG):	2,112	2,970	3,704	3,997
CALCIUM (MG):	939	1,045	1,107	1,250
% CARB	43	43	43	43
% PROTEIN	27	27	28	27
% FAT	30	30	29	30

Daily Calorie Level	1,200	1,500	1,800	2,100
BREAKFAST	½ cup (dry measure) oatmeal with 1 TBSP dried apricots 1 cup nonfat or low-fat milk	½ cup (dry measure) oatmeal with 2 TBSP each dried apricots and pecans 1 cup nonfat or low-fat milk 1 hard-boiled egg	⅔ cup (dry measure) oatmeal with 2 TBSP each dried apricots and pecans 1 cup nonfat or low-fat milk 1 hard-boiled egg	⅔ cup (dry measure) oatmeal with 2 TBSP each dried apricots and pecans 1 cup nonfat or low-fat milk 1 hard-boiled egg
LUNCH	1¼ cups Cranberry-Crunch Chicken Salad (p. 158) over mixed salad greens with 1 TBSP light balsamic vinaigrette	1½ cups Cranberry-Crunch Chicken Salad (p. 158) over mixed salad greens with 1 TBSP light balsamic vinaigrette	1½ cups Cranberry-Crunch Chicken Salad (p. 158) over mixed salad greens with 1 TBSP light balsamic vinaigrette	1¾ cups Cranberry-Crunch Chicken Salad (p. 158) over mixed salad greens with 1 TBSP light balsamic vinaigrette
SNACK	¼ cup Scallion & Olive Hummus (p. 136) 2 stalks celery	⅓ cup Scallion & Olive Hummus (p. 136) 6 whole grain crackers	⅓ cup Scallion & Olive Hummus (p. 136) 6 whole grain crackers	⅓ cup Scallion & Olive Hummus (p. 136) 6 whole grain crackers
DINNER	Lazy-Day Lasagna (p. 198) Sicilian-style Asparagus (p. 169) Side salad with 1 TBSP light olive oil vinaigrette	Lazy-Day Lasagna (p. 198) Sicilian-style Asparagus (p. 169) Side salad with 1 TBSP light olive oil vinaigrette	Lazy-Day Lasagna (p. 198) Sicilian-style Asparagus (p. 169) Side salad with 1 TBSP light olive oil vinaigrette	1½ servings Lazy-Day Lasagna (p. 198) Sicilian-style Asparagus (p. 169) Side salad with 1 TBSP light olive oil vinaigrette

DINNER *(continued)*			Chocolate-Peanut Butter Parfait (p. 225)	Chocolate-Peanut Butter Parfait (p. 225)
TOTAL CALORIES:	1,166	1,505	1,768	1,993
CARBS (G):	131	163	200	221
FAT (G):	37	54	61	67
SAT. FAT (G):	8.8	10.3	11.8	14.5
CHOL. (MG):	104	304	306	338
PROTEIN (G):	84	97	107	127
FIBER (G):	22	27	30	31
SODIUM (MG):	1,792	2,040	2,266	2,635
CALCIUM (MG):	1,179	1,141	1,316	1,597
% CARB	44	43	45	44
% PROTEIN	28	25	24	26
% FAT	28	32	31	30

Daily Calorie Level	1,200	1,500	1,800	2,100
BREAKFAST	¾ cup nonfat or low-fat cottage cheese in a cantaloupe half 2 TBSP walnuts	¾ cup nonfat or low-fat cottage cheese in a cantaloupe half 2 TBSP walnuts	1 cup nonfat or low-fat cottage cheese in a cantaloupe half 3 TBSP walnuts	1 cup nonfat or low-fat cottage cheese in a cantaloupe half 3 TBSP walnuts
LUNCH	1½ cups Slow-cooked Beef, Barley, & Vegetable Soup (p. 142) 1 medium sliced apple spread with 1 TBSP peanut butter	2 cups Slow-cooked Beef, Barley, & Vegetable Soup (p. 142) 1 medium sliced apple spread with 1 TBSP peanut butter	2 cups Slow-cooked Beef, Barley, & Vegetable Soup (p. 142) ½ egg salad sandwich on whole-wheat bread 1 large sliced apple spread with 1 TBSP peanut butter	2 cups Slow-cooked Beef, Barley, & Vegetable Soup (p. 142) 1 egg salad sandwich on whole-wheat bread 1 large sliced apple spread with 1 TBSP peanut butter
SNACK	8 ounces light yogurt	8 ounces light yogurt ¼ cup low-fat granola	8 ounces light yogurt ¼ cup low-fat granola	8 ounces light yogurt ¼ cup low-fat granola
DINNER	Grecian-style Grouper (p. 215) ½ cup Mediterranean White Bean Salad (p. 165)	Grecian-style Grouper (p. 215) 1 cup Mediterranean White Bean Salad (p. 165)	Grecian-style Grouper (p. 215) 1 cup Mediterranean White Bean Salad (p. 165)	Grecian-style Grouper (p. 215) 1 cup Mediterranean White Bean Salad (p. 165)

DINNER *(continued)*	⅔ cup Easy Oven-baked Vegetables (p. 170)	1 cup Easy Oven-baked Vegetables (p. 170)	1 cup Easy Oven-baked Vegetables (p. 170)	1 cup Easy Oven-baked Vegetables (p. 170) I cup low-fat ice cream
TOTAL CALORIES:	1,183	1,448	1,756	2,105
CARBS (G):	125	170	196	239
FAT (G):	35	42	59	73
SAT. FAT (G):	6	6.8	9.4	13
CHOL. (MG):	120	135	217	302
PROTEIN (G):	100	115	129	140
FIBER (G):	21	30	34	37
SODIUM (MG):	2,345	2,962	3,451	3,831
CALCIUM (MG):	727	804	878	1,064
% CARB	41	45	43	44
% PROTEIN	33	30	28	26
% FAT	26	25	29	30

Daily Calorie Level	1,200	1,500	1,800	2,100
BREAKFAST	Primavera Omelette (p. 118) 2 slices turkey bacon 1 cup mixed fresh fruit	Primavera Omelette (p. 118) 2 slices turkey bacon 1 cup mixed fresh fruit	Primavera Omelette (p. 118) 2 slices turkey bacon 1 cup mixed fresh fruit	Primavera Omelet (p. 118) 2 slices turkey bacon 1 cup mixed fresh fruit 1 cup nonfat or low-fat milk
LUNCH	Salad Niçoise (p. 156)	Salad Niçoise (p. 156) 1 cup Butterbean Soup (p. 150)	Salad Niçoise (p. 156) 1 cup Butterbean Soup (p. 150)	Salad Niçoise (p. 156) 1 cup Butterbean Soup (p. 150)
SNACK	½ peanut butter & banana sandwich on whole wheat 1 cup nonfat or low-fat milk	½ peanut butter & banana sandwich on whole wheat 1 cup nonfat or low-fat milk	1 peanut butter & banana sandwich on whole wheat 1 cup nonfat or low-fat milk	1 peanut butter & banana sandwich on whole wheat 1 cup nonfat or low-fat milk
DINNER	2 Spicy Chicken Enchiladas (p. 207) ½ cup Cilantro-Carrot Salad (p. 164) ⅔ cup sautéed zucchini & onions	2 Spicy Chicken Enchiladas (p. 207) ½ cup Cilantro-Carrot Salad (p. 164) ⅔ cup sautéed zucchini & onions	2 Spicy Chicken Enchiladas (p. 207) ½ cup Cilantro-Carrot Salad (p. 164) ⅔ cup sautéed zucchini & onions	3 Spicy Chicken Enchiladas (p. 207) ½ cup Cilantro-Carrot Salad (p. 164) ⅔ cup sautéed zucchini & onions

DINNER (continued)		2 TBSP chocolate-covered almonds	3 TBSP chocolate-covered almonds	⅓ cup chocolate-covered almonds
TOTAL CALORIES:	1,186	1,483	1,770	2,078
CARBS (G):	128	166	202	232
FAT (G):	39	50	64	77
SAT. FAT (G):	7.6	9.6	11.8	14.5
CHOL. (MG):	276	291	291	311
PROTEIN (G):	90	107	116	135
FIBER (G):	19	30	35	38
SODIUM (MG):	2,241	2,596	2,801	3,112
CALCIUM (MG):	851	937	1,000	1,443
% CARB	42	43	44	43
% PROTEIN	29	28	25	25
% FAT	29	29	31	32

Daily Calorie Level	1,200	1,500	1,800	2,100
BREAKFAST	¾ cup high-fiber cereal ½ cup blueberries 1 cup nonfat or low-fat milk 1 hard-boiled egg	1 cup high-fiber cereal ½ cup blueberries 1 cup nonfat or low-fat milk 1 hard-boiled egg	1 cup high-fiber cereal ½ cup blueberries 1 cup nonfat or low-fat milk 1 hard-boiled egg Vegetarian sausage patty	1 cup high-fiber cereal ½ cup blueberries 1 cup nonfat or low-fat milk 1 hard-boiled egg Vegetarian sausage patty
LUNCH	Unfried Fish Sandwich on a light wheat bun (p. 181) ¾ cup Broccoli Slaw (p. 166)	Unfried Fish Sandwich on a light wheat bun (p. 181) ¾ cup Broccoli Slaw (p. 166) 1 cup nonfat or low-fat milk	Unfried Fish Sandwich on a light wheat bun (p. 181) ¾ cup Broccoli Slaw (p. 166) 1 cup nonfat or low-fat milk	Unfried Fish Sandwich on a multigrain bun (p. 181) ¾ cup Broccoli Slaw (p. 166) 1 cup nonfat or low-fat milk
SNACK	½ cup cottage cheese 1 canned peach half in juice	¾ cup cottage cheese 1 canned peach half in juice 2 tablespoons pecans	¾ cup cottage cheese 2 canned peach halves in juice ¼ cup pecans	¾ cup cottage cheese 2 canned peach halves in juice ¼ cup pecans
DINNER	4 ounces Seared Cajun Chicken (p. 208)	4 ounces Seared Cajun Chicken (p. 208)	4 ounces Seared Cajun Chicken (p. 208)	5 ounces Seared Cajun Chicken (p. 208)

DINNER (continued)	Cranberry-Apple Spinach Salad (p. 165) Small baked sweet potato with 1 tsp trans-free margarine	Cranberry-Apple Spinach Salad (p. 165) Small baked sweet potato with 1 tsp trans-free margarine	Cranberry-Apple Spinach Salad (p. 165) Medium baked sweet potato with 1½ tsp trans-free margarine	Cranberry-Apple Spinach Salad (p. 165) Medium baked sweet potato with 1½ tsp trans-free margarine Cherry Fudge Cake (p. 222)
TOTAL CALORIES:	1,143	1,461	1,760	2,042
CARBS (G):	130	158	188	227
FAT (G):	31	45	60	66
SAT. FAT (G):	5.5	7.3	9.1	10.8
CHOL. (MG):	335	371	371	397
PROTEIN (G):	93	119	132	145
FIBER (G):	21	24	30	33
SODIUM (MG):	2,008	2,446	2,751	3,223
CALCIUM (MG):	609	963	995	1,075
% CARB	45	42	41	44
% PROTEIN	31	31	29	28
% FAT	23	27	30	28

Daily Calorie Level	1,200	1,500	1,800	2,100
BREAKFAST	Southwestern Egg Sandwich (p. 122) 1 cup honeydew melon	Southwestern Egg Sandwich (p. 122) 1 cup honeydew melon 1 cup nonfat or low-fat milk	Southwestern Egg Sandwich (p. 122) 1 cup honeydew melon 1 cup nonfat or low-fat milk	Southwestern Egg Sandwich (p. 122) 1 cup honeydew melon 1 cup nonfat or low-fat milk
LUNCH	Rotisserie Chicken Salad (p. 155)	Rotisserie Chicken Salad (p. 155) 1 cup canned reduced-sodium bean soup	Rotisserie Chicken Salad (p. 155) 1 cup canned reduced-sodium bean soup	Rotisserie Chicken Salad (p. 155) 1½ cups canned reduced-sodium bean soup
SNACK	1 oz low-fat cheese Medium pear	1 oz low-fat cheese Medium pear	1 oz low-fat cheese Medium pear 3 TBSP walnuts	1½ oz low-fat cheese Large pear ¼ cup walnuts
DINNER	3 oz Grilled Tuscan Tenderloin (p. 214) Herb-roasted Corn (p. 173) ⅔ cup Green Beans with Almonds (p. 171) Sliced fresh tomatoes	4 oz Grilled Tuscan Tenderloin (p. 214) Herb-roasted Corn (p. 173) ⅔ cup Green Beans with Almonds (p. 171) Sliced fresh tomatoes	4 oz Grilled Tuscan Tenderloin (p. 214) Herb-roasted Corn (p. 173) ⅔ cup Green Beans with Almonds (p. 171) Sliced fresh tomatoes	5 oz Grilled Tuscan Tenderloin (p. 214) Herb-roasted Corn (p. 173) 1 cup Green Beans with Almonds (p. 171) Sliced fresh tomatoes

DINNER *(continued)*			Sensational Berry Sundaes (p. 230)	Sensational Berry Sundaes (p. 230)
TOTAL CALORIES:	1,174	1,462	1,763	2,057
CARBS (G):	118	158	190	221
FAT (G):	39	43	61	72
SAT. FAT (G):	8.6	10	12	15
CHOL. (MG):	176	208	213	245
PROTEIN (G):	94	121	130	150
FIBER (G):	20	25	29	36
SODIUM (MG):	2,000	2,695	2,765	3,256
CALCIUM (MG):	926	1,311	1,453	1,662
% CARB	40	42	42	41
% PROTEIN	31	32	28	28
% FAT	29	26	30	31

Daily Calorie Level	1,200	1,500	1,800	2,100
BREAKFAST	Zucchini-Onion Frittata (p. 119) ½ grapefruit 1 cup nonfat or low-fat milk	Zucchini-Onion Frittata (p. 119) ½ grapefruit 1 cup nonfat or low-fat milk 2 oz low-fat smoked sausage	Zucchini-Onion Frittata (p. 119) ½ grapefruit 1 cup nonfat or low-fat milk 2 oz low-fat smoked sausage	1½ servings Zucchini-Onion Frittata (p. 119) ½ grapefruit 1 cup nonfat or low-fat milk 2 oz low-fat smoked sausage
LUNCH	Veggie burger with low-fat cheese and veggie trimmings on a light wheat bun Cup of tomato soup	Veggie burger with low-fat cheese and veggie trimmings on a multigrain bun Cup of tomato soup	Veggie burger with low-fat cheese and veggie trimmings on a multigrain bun Cup of black bean soup	Veggie burger with low-fat cheese and veggie trimmings on a multigrain bun Cup of black bean soup ½ cup nonfat or low-fat cottage cheese
SNACK	2 stalks celery filled with 2 TBSP peanut butter	2 stalks celery filled with 2 TBSP peanut butter	2 stalks celery filled with 2 TBSP peanut butter	2 stalks celery filled with 3 TBSP peanut butter
DINNER	Stuffed Chicken Breast Florentine (p. 203) Broiled Asparagus (p. 169)	Stuffed Chicken Breast Florentine (p. 203) 1 cup Summer Garden Pilaf (p. 174)	Stuffed Chicken Breast Florentine (p. 203) 1 cup Summer Garden Pilaf (p. 174)	Stuffed Chicken Breast Florentine (p. 203) 1 cup Summer Garden Pilaf (p. 174)

DINNER (continued)	Side salad with 2 TBSP light Italian dressing	Side salad with 2 TBSP light Italian dressing	Side salad with 2 TBSP light Italian dressing 2 Chocolate Chip- Raisin Cookies (p. 227) with 1 cup nonfat or low-fat milk	Side salad with 2 TBSP light Italian dressing 3 Chocolate Chip- Raisin Cookies (p. 227) with 1 cup nonfat or low-fat milk
TOTAL CALORIES:	1,201	1,460	1,771	2,079
CARBS (G):	124	159	203	225
FAT (G):	40	47	57	71
SAT. FAT (G):	6	7.3	9.4	12.9
CHOL. (MG):	105	159	133	154
PROTEIN (G):	96	105	122	150
FIBER (G):	27	25	35	40
SODIUM (MG):	2,750	3,296	3,769	4,392
CALCIUM (MG):	918	935	1,295	1,576
% CARB	40	43	45	42
% PROTEIN	31	28	27	28
% FAT	29	29	29	30

Daily Calorie Level	1,200	1,500	1,800	2,100
BREAKFAST	Poached egg on whole-grain toast 1 cup nonfat or low-fat milk 1 cup mixed fresh berries	Poached egg on whole-grain toast 1 cup nonfat or low-fat milk 1 cup mixed fresh berries	Poached egg on whole-grain toast 1 cup nonfat or low-fat milk 1 cup mixed fresh berries Vegetarian sausage patty	Poached egg on whole-grain toast 1 cup nonfat or low-fat milk 1 cup mixed fresh berries Vegetarian sausage patty
LUNCH	Chicken Gyros (p. 180)	Chicken Gyros (p. 180) Cup of bean soup	Chicken Gyros (p. 180) Cup of bean soup	Chicken Gyros (p. 180) 1½ cups bean soup
SNACK	6 oz V8 juice 3 TBSP roasted peanuts	6 oz V8 juice ¼ cup roasted peanuts 1 ounce low-fat cheese	6 oz V8 juice ⅓ cup roasted peanuts 1 ounce low-fat cheese	6 oz V8 juice ⅓ cup roasted peanuts 1 ounce low-fat cheese
DINNER	Pork Tenderloin with Butternut Squash & Onions (p. 212) ⅔ cup Spinach & Onion Sauté (p. 177) Summer Tomato Salad (p. 164)	Pork Tenderloin with Butternut Squash & Onions (p. 212) ⅔ cup Spinach & Onion Sauté (p. 177) Summer Tomato Salad (p. 164)	Pork Tenderloin with Butternut Squash & Onions (p. 212) ⅔ cup Spinach & Onion Sauté (p. 177) Summer Tomato Salad (p. 164)	1½ servings Pork Tenderloin with Butternut Squash & Onions (p. 212) ⅔ cup Spinach & Onion Sauté (p. 177) Summer Tomato Salad (p. 164)

DINNER *(continued)*			Cinnamon-Peach Crisp (p. 229)	Cinnamon-Peach Crisp (p. 229) with ½ cup low-fat vanilla ice cream
TOTAL CALORIES:	1,157	1,440	1,752	2,045
CARBS (G):	122	151	184	224
FAT (G):	39	50	64	71
SAT. FAT (G):	7.7	10.8	13	15.2
CHOL. (MG):	330	351	351	392
PROTEIN (G):	92	114	131	152
FIBER (G):	25	30	36	42
SODIUM (MG):	1,875	2,577	3,047	3,509
CALCIUM (MG):	931	1,273	1,321	1,579
% CARB	41	40	40	42
% PROTEIN	30	30	29	28
% FAT	29	30	31	30

Daily Calorie Level	1,200	1,500	1,800	2,100
BREAKFAST	Southwestern Egg Scramble (p. 121) 2 oz turkey sausage ¾ cup diced mangoes and blueberries 1 cup nonfat or low-fat milk	Southwestern Egg Scramble (p. 121) 2 oz turkey sausage 1 cup diced mangoes and blueberries 1 cup nonfat or low-fat milk	1½ servings Southwestern Egg Scramble (p. 121) 2 oz turkey sausage 1 cup diced mangoes and blueberries 1 cup nonfat or low-fat milk	1½ servings Southwestern Egg Scramble (p. 121) 2 oz turkey sausage 1 cup diced mangoes and blueberries 1 cup nonfat or low-fat milk
LUNCH	Tempting Turkey Wraps (p. 184)	Tempting Turkey Wraps (p. 184) ⅔ cup Light Carrot-Raisin Salad (p.163)	Tempting Turkey Wraps (p. 184) ⅔ cup Light Carrot-Raisin Salad (p. 163)	Tempting Turkey Wraps (p. 184) 1 cup canned lentil soup ⅔ cup Light Carrot-Raisin Salad (p. 163)
SNACK	¾ cup grapes 1 oz low-fat cheese	¾ cup grapes 1 oz low-fat cheese 3 TBSP walnuts	1 cup grapes 1½ oz low-fat cheese ¼ cup walnuts	1 cup grapes 1½ oz low-fat cheese ⅓ cup walnuts
DINNER	Meat & Potato Pie (p. 210) Spinach & Mushroom Salad (p. 162)	Meat & Potato Pie (p. 210) Spinach & Mushroom Salad (p. 162)	1½ servings Meat & Potato Pie (p. 210) Spinach & Mushroom Salad (p. 162)	1½ servings Meat & Potato Pie (p. 210) Spinach & Mushroom Salad (p. 162) 1 ounce dark chocolate

TOTAL CALORIES:	1,229	1,444	1,756	2,069
CARBS (G):	129	153	181	215
FAT (G):	35	48	58	76
SAT. FAT (G):	11.3	12.5	15.5	22.6
CHOL. (MG):	276	276	310	310
PROTEIN (G):	99	103	130	141
FIBER (G):	14	18	22	28
SODIUM (MG):	2,459	2,590	3,219	3,662
CALCIUM (MG):	978	1,027	1,274	1,340
% CARB	42	42	41	41
% PROTEIN	32	28	29	27
% FAT	26	29	30	32

Daily Calorie Level	1,200	1,500	1,800	2,100
BREAKFAST	Ham & Pepper Frittata (p. 120) 1 cup mixed fresh fruit 1 cup nonfat or low-fat milk	Ham & Pepper Frittata (p. 120) 1 cup mixed fresh fruit 1 cup nonfat or low-fat milk	1½ servings Ham & Pepper Frittata (p. 120) 1 cup mixed fresh fruit 1 cup nonfat or low-fat milk	1½ servings Ham & Pepper Frittata (p. 120) 1 cup mixed fresh fruit 1 cup nonfat or low-fat milk
LUNCH	2 cups Southwestern Chicken Soup (p. 143)	2 cups Southwestern Chicken Soup (p. 143) Fresh vegetables with 2 TBSP light ranch dressing	2 cups Southwestern Chicken Soup (p. 143) Fresh vegetables with 2 TBSP light ranch dressing	2 cups Southwestern Chicken Soup (p. 143) Fresh vegetables with 2 TBSP light ranch dressing
SNACK	2 TBSP mixed nuts	1 oz low-fat cheese 2 TBSP mixed nuts	1 oz low-fat cheese 3 TBSP mixed nuts	1 oz low-fat cheese ¼ cup mixed nuts Medium apple
DINNER	1¾ cups Penne with Sausage, Peppers, & Onions (p. 191) Side salad with 1 TBSP light Italian dressing	2 cups Penne with Sausage, Peppers, & Onions (p. 191) Side salad with 1 TBSP light Italian dressing	2 cups Penne with Sausage, Peppers, & Onions (p. 191) Side salad with 1 TBSP light Italian dressing Baked Pears with Citrus Sauce (p. 229)	2½ cups Penne with Sausage, Peppers, & Onions (p. 191) Side salad with 1 TBSP light Italian dressing

DINNER (continued)				Baked Pears with Citrus Sauce (p. 229)
TOTAL CALORIES:	1,228	1,511	1,833	2,080
CARBS (G):	125	151	188	226
FAT (G):	38	51	64	72
SAT. FAT (G):	8.9	12	14.3	15
CHOL. (MG):	161	195	211	211
PROTEIN (G):	95	112	128	137
FIBER (G):	20	23	27	33
SODIUM (MG):	2,776	3,398	3,822	3,834
CALCIUM (MG):	821	1,119	1,295	1,325
% CARB	41	40	41	43
% PROTEIN	31	30	28	26
% FAT	28	30	31	31
% ALCOHOL				7

References

CHAPTER 1

1. American Diabetes Association and National Institute of Diabetes, Digestive, and Kidney Disease. The prevention or delay of type 2 diabetes. *Diabetes Care.* 2002;25(4):742–49.

2. Boyle, J. P., A. A. Honeycutt, K. M. Venkat Narayan, T. J. Hoerger, L. S. Geiss, H. Chen, and T. J. Thompson. Projection of diabetes burden through 2050. *Diabetes Care.* 2001;24:1936–40.

3. Centers for Disease Control. National Diabetes Fact Sheet *http://www.cdc.gov/diabetes/pubs/estimates. htm* (accessed 3/24/03).

4. Convit, A., O. T. Wolf, C. Tarshish, and M. J. de Leon. Reduced glucose tolerance is associated with poor memory performance and hippocampal atrophy among normal elderly. Proceedings of the National Academy of Sciences. 2003;100(4):2019–22.

5. Fagot-Campagna, A. Emergence of type 2 diabetes mellitus in children: epidemiological evidence. *Journal of Pediatric Endocrinology and Metabolism.* 2000;13(suppl 6):1395–1402.

6. Ford, E.S., W. H. Giles, and W. H. Dietz. Prevalence of the metabolic syndrome among US adults. *Journal of the American Medical Association.* 2002;287:356–59.

7. Lakka, H. M., D. E. Laaksonen, T. A. Lakka, L. K. Niskanen, K. Esko, J. Tuomilehto, and J. T. Salonen. The metabolic syndrome and total and cardiovascular disease mortality in middle-aged men. *Journal of the American Medical Association.* 2002;288(21):2708–16.

8. Minehira, K., and L. Tappy. Dietary and lifestyle interventions in the management of the metabolic syndrome: present status and future perspective. *European Journal of Clinical Nutrition.* 2002;56(12): 1264–69.

9. National Institute of Diabetes and Digestive and Kidney Diseases. *Am I at Risk for Diabetes?* NIH publication No. 02-4805; May 2002. (Accessed 12/8/02 at *http://www.niddk.nih.gov/health/diabetes/pubs/ risk/risk.htm#7*).

10. National Institutes of Health, National Heart, Lung, and Blood Institute. Third Report of the National Cholesterol Education Program Expert Panel on Detection, Evaluation, and Treatment of High Blood Cholesterol in Adults (Adult Treatment Panel III). NIH Publication 02-5215; September 2002.

11. Siedell, J. C. Obesity, insulin resistance, and diabetes—a worldwide epidemic. *British Journal of Nutrition.* 2000;83(suppl 1):S5–S8.
12. Sinha, R., G. Fisch, B. Teague, W. V. Tamborlane, B. Banyas, K. Allen, M. Savoye, V. Rieger, S. Taksali, G. Barbetta, R. S. Sherwin, and S. Caprio. Prevalence of impaired glucose tolerance among children and adolescents with marked obesity. *New England Journal of Medicine.* 2002;346(11):802–10.

CHAPTER 2

1. Chaisson, J. L., R. G. Josse, R. Gomis, M. Hanefeld, A. Karaski, M. Laakso; STOP-NIDDM Trail Research Group. Acarbose for prevention of type 2 diabetes mellitus: the STOP-NIDDM randomised trial. *Lancet* 2002;359(9323):2072–77.
2. The Diabetes Prevention Program (DPP) Research Group. Reduction in the incidence of type 2 diabetes with lifestyle intervention or metformin. *New England Journal of Medicine.* 2002;346:393–403.
3. The Diabetes Prevention Program (DPP) Research Group. The Diabetes Prevention Program: Description of lifestyle intervention. *Diabetes Care.* 2002;25:2165–71.
4. Eriksson, K. F. and F. Lindgarde. Prevention of type 2 (noninsulin-dependent) diabetes mellitus by diet and physical exercise. The 6-year Malmo feasibility study. *Diabetologia.* 1991;34(12):891–98.
5. Hu, F. B., J. E. Manson, M. J. Stampfer, G. Colditz, S. Liu, C. G. Solomon, and W. C. Willett. Diet, lifestyle, and the risk of type 2 diabetes mellitus in women. *New England Journal of Medicine.* 2001;345:790–97.
6. Pan, X. R., G. W. Li, Y. H. Hu, J. X. Wang, W. Y. Yang, Z. X. An, J. Lin, J. Z. Xiao, H. B. Cao, P. A. Liu, X. G. Jiang, Y. Y. Jiang, J. P. Wang, H. Zheng, H. Zhang, P. H. Bennett, and B. V. Howard. Effects of diet and exercise in preventing NIDDM in people with impaired glucose tolerance. The Da Qing IGT and diabetes study. *Diabetes Care.* 1997;20(4):537–44.
7. Tuomillehto, J., J. Lindstrom, J. G. Eriksson, T. T. Valle, H. Hamalainen, P. Ilanne-Parikka, S. Keinanen-Kiukaanniemi, M. Laakso, A. Louheranta, M. Rastas, V. Salminen, and M. Uusitupa. Prevention of type 2 diabetes mellitus by changes in lifestyle among subjects with impaired glucose tolerance. *New England Journal of Medicine.* 2001;344:1343–50.

CHAPTER 3

1. Chan, J. M., E. B. Rimm, G. A. Colditz, M. J. Stampfer, and W. C. Willett. Obesity, fat distribution, and weight gain as risk factors for clinical diabetes in men. *Diabetes Care.* 1994;17(9): 961–69.
2. Chrousos, G. P. The role of stress and the hypothalamic pituitary-adrenal axis in the pathogenesis of the metabolic syndrome: neuro-endocrine and target tissue-related causes. *International Journal of Obesity.* 2000;24(suppl 2):S50–S55.
3. Colditz, G. A., W. C. Willet, M. J. Stampfer, J. E. Manson, C. H. Hennekens, R. A. Arky, and F. E. Speizer. Weight as a risk factor for clinical diabetes in women. *American Journal of Epidemiology.* 1990;132(3):501–13.
4. Colditz, G. A., W. C. Willet, A. Rotnitzky, and J. E. Manson. Weight gain as a risk factor for clinical diabetes mellitus in women. *Annals of Internal Medicine.* 1995;122(7):548–49.
5. Field, A. E., E. H. Coakley, A. Must, J. L. Spadano, N. Laird, W. H. Dietz, E. Rimm, and G. A. Colditz.

Impact of overweight on the risk of developing common chronic diseases during a 10-year period. *Archives of Internal Medicine.* 2001;161:1581–86.

6. Hill, J. O., and R. R. Wing. Successful weight loss maintenance. *Annual Review of Nutrition.* 2001; 21:323–41.

7. Klem, M. L., R. R. Wing, W. Lang, M. T. McGuire, and J. O. Hill. Does weight maintenance become easier over time? *Obesity Research.* 2000;8(6):438–44.

8. Knight, E. L., M. J. Stampfer, S. E. Hankinson, D. Spiegelman, and G. C. Curhan. The impact of protein intake on renal function decline in women with normal renal function or mild renal insufficiency. *Annals of Internal Medicine.* 2003;138(6):460–67.

9. Layman, D. K., R. A. Boileau, D. J. Erickson, J. E. Painter, H. Shiue, C. Sather, and D. D. Christou. A reduced ratio of dietary carbohydrate to protein improves body composition and blood lipid profiles during weight loss in adult women. *Journal of Nutrition.* 2003;133:411–17.

10. Layman, D. K., H. Shiue, C. Sather, D. J. Erikson, and J. Baum. Increased dietary protein modifies glucose and insulin homeostasis in adult women during weight loss. *Journal of Nutrition.* 2003;133:405–10.

11. McCrory, M. A., P. J. Fuss, J. E. McCallum, M. Yao, A. G. Vinken, N. P. Hays, and S. B. Roberts. Dietary variety within food groups: association with energy intake and body fatness in men and women. *American Journal of Clinical Nutrition.* 1999;69:440–47.

12. Rolls, B. J., E. Morris, and L. S. Roe. Portion size of food affects energy intake in normal-weight and overweight men and women. *American Journal of Clinical Nutrition.* 2002; 76(6):1207–13.

13. Schlundt, D. G., J. O. Hill, T. Sbrocco, J. Pope-Cordle, and T. Sharp. The role of breakfast in the treatment of obesity: a randomized clinical trial. *American Journal of Clinical Nutrition.* 1992;55(3):645–51.

14. Skov, A. R., S. Toubro, B. Ronn, L. Holm, and A. Astrup. Randomized trial on protein vs carbohydrate in ad libitum fat reduced diet for the treatment of obesity. *International Journal of Obesity.* 1999;23:528–36.

15. Serdula, M. K., A. H. Mokdad, D. F. Williamson, D. A. Galuska, J. M. Mendlein, and G. W. Heath. Prevalence of attempting weight loss and strategies for controlling weight. *Journal of the American Medical Association.* 1999;282:1353–58.

16. Spiegal, K., R. Leproult, and E. Van Cauter. Impact of sleep debt on metabolic and endocrine function. *Lancet.* 1999;354:1435–39.

17. Van Cauter, E., R. Leproult, and L. Plat. Age-related changes in slow wave sleep and REM sleep and relationship with growth hormone and cortisol levels in healthy men. *Journal of the American Medical Association.* 2000;284(7):861–68.

18. Wing, R. R., G. K. Grunwald, C. L. Mosea, M. L. Klem, and J. O. Hill. Long-term weight loss and breakfast in subjects in the national weight control registry. *Obesity Research.* 2002;10(2):78–82.

19. Young, L. R., and M. Nestle. The contribution of expanding portion sizes to the US obesity epidemic. *American Journal of Public Health.* 2002;92:246–49.

CHAPTER 4

1. Ajani, U. A., C. H. Hennekens, A. Spelsberg, and J. E. Manson. Alcohol consumption and risk of type 2 diabetes mellitus among US male physicians. *Archives of Internal Medicine.* 2000; 160(7):1025–30.

2. Chandalia, M., A. Garg, D. Lutjohann, K. von Bergmann, S. M. Grundy, and L. J. Brinkley. Beneficial effects of high dietary fiber intake in patients with type 2 diabetes melliutus. *New England Journal of Medicine.* 2000;342:1392–98.

3. Davies, M. J., D. J. Baer, J. T. Judd, E. D. Brown, W. S. Campbell, and P. R. Taylor. Effects of moderate alcohol intake on fasting insulin and glucose concentrations and insulin sensitivity in postmenopausal women: a randomized controlled trial. *Journal of the American Medical Association.* 2002;287(19):2559–2562.

4. Foster-Powell, K., S. H. A. Holt, and J. C. Brand-Miller. International table of glycemic index and glycemic load values: *American Journal of Clinical Nutrition.* 2002;76:5–56.

5. Fung, T. T., F. B. Hu, M. A. Pereira, S. Liu, M. J. Stampfer, G. A. Colditz, and W. C. Willett. Whole-grain intake and the risk of type 2 diabetes: a prospective study in men. *American Journal of Clinical Nutrition.* 2002;(3):535–40.

6. Hu, F. B., R. M. van Dam, and S. Liu. Diet and risk of type 2 diabetes: the role of types of fat and carbohydrate. *Diabetologia.* 2001;44:805–17.

7. Jarvi, A. E., B. E. Karlstrom, Y. Granfeldt, I. Bjorck, N. L. Asp, and B. Vessby. Improved glycemic control and lipid profile and normalized fibrinolytic activity on a low-glycemic index diet in type 2 diabetic patients. *Diabetes Care.* 1999;22(1):10–18.

8. Jiang, R., J. E. Manson, M. J. Stampfer, S. Liu, W. C. Willett, and F. B. Hu. Nut and peanut butter consumption and risk of type 2 diabetes in women. *Journal of the American Medical Association.* 2002; 288(20):2554–60.

9. Liu, S., J. E. Manson, M. J. Stampfer, F. B. Hu, E. Giovannucci, G. A. Colditz, C. H. Hennekens, and W. C. Willet. A prospective study of whole-grain intake and risk of type 2 diabetes mellitus in US women. *American Journal of Public Health.* 2000;90(9):1409–15.

10. Ludwig, D. S. The glycemic index: Physiological mechanisms relating to obesity, diabetes, and cardiovascular disease. *Journal of the American Medical Association.* 2002;287:2414–23.

11. Luscombe, N. D., M. Noakes, and P. M. Clifton. Diets high and low in glycemic index versus high monounsaturated fat diets: effect on glucose and lipid metabolism in NIDDM. *European Journal of Clinical Nutrition.* 1999;53:473–78.

12. McKeown, N. M., J. B. Meigs, S. Liu, W. F. Wilson, and P. F. Jacques. Whole-grain intake is favorably associated with metabolic risk factors for type 2 diabetes and cardiovascular disease in the Framingham Offspring Study. *American Journal of Clinical Nutrition.* 2002;76:390–98.

13. Meyer, K. A., L. H. Kushi, D. R. Jacobs, and A. R. Folsom. Dietary fat and incidence of type 2 diabetes in older Iowa women. *Diabetes Care.* 2001;(9):1528–35.

14. Meyer, K. A., L. H. Kushi, D. R. Jacobs Jr, J. Slavin, T. A. Sellers, and A. R. Folsom. Carbohydrates, dietary fiber, and incident type 2 diabetes in older women. *American Journal of Clinical Nutrition.* 2000;(4):921–30.

15. Montonen, J., P. Knekt, R. Jarvinen, A. Aromaa, and Reunanen Antti. Whole grain and fiber intake and the incidence of type 2 diabetes. *American Journal of Clinical Nutrition.* 2003;77(3):622–29.

16. Salmeron, J., A. Ascherio, E. B. Rimm, G. A. Colditz, D. Spiegelman, D. J. Jenkins, M. J. Stampfer, A. L. Wing, and W. C. Willett. Dietary fiber, glycemic load, and risk of NIDDM in men. *Diabetes Care.* 1997;(4):545–50.

17. Salmeron, J., F. B. Hu, J. E. Manson, M. J. Stampfer, G. A. Colditz, E. B. Rimm, and W. C. Willett. Dietary fat intake and risk of type 2 diabetes in women. *American Journal of Clinical Nutrition.* 2001;(6):1019–26.

18. Salmeron, J., J. E. Manson, M. J. Stampfer, G. A. Colditz, A. L. Wing, and W. C. Willett. Dietary fiber, glycemic load, and risk of non-insulin-dependent diabetes mellitus in women. *Journal of the American Medical Association.* 1997;277(6):472–77.

19. Simopoulos, A. P. Essential fatty acids in health and chronic disease. *American Journal of Clinical Nutrition.* 1999;70(suppl):560S–69S.
20. Van Dam, R. M., E. B. Rimm, W. C. Willett, M. J. Stampfer, and F. B. Hu. Dietary patterns and risk for type 2 diabetes mellitus in U.S. men. *Annals of Internal Medicine.* 2002;136(3):201–09.

CHAPTER 5

1. Heaney, R. P., K. M. Davies, and J. Barger-Lux. Calcium and weight: clinical studies. *Journal of the American College of Nutrition.* 2002;21(2):152S–55S.
2. Jiang, R., J. E. Manson, M. J. Stampfer, W. C. Willett, and F. B. Hu. Nut and peanut butter consumption and risk of type 2 diabetes in women. *Journal of the American Medical Association.* 2002; 288(20):2554–60.
3. Kris-Etherton, P. M., W. S. Harris, and L. J. Appel. AHA Scientific Statement: Fish consumption, fish oil, omega-3 fatty acids, and cardiovascular disease. *Circulation.* 2002;106:2747–57.
4. Montonen, J., P. Knekt, R. Jarvinen, A. Aromaa, and A. Reunanen. Whole grain and fiber intake and the incidence of type 2 diabetes. *American Journal of Clinical Nutrition.* 2003;77(3):622–29.
5. Periera, M. A., D. R. Jacobs, J. J. Pins, S. K. Raatz, M. D. Gross, J. L. Slavin, and E. R. Seaquist. Effect of whole grains on insulin sensitivity in overweight hyperinsulinemic adults. *American Journal of Clinical Nutrition.* 2002;75:848–55.

CHAPTER 6

1. French, S. A., L. Harnack, and R. W. Jeffrey. Fast food restaurant use among women in the Pound of Prevention study: dietary, behavioral and demographic correlates. *International Journal of Obesity.* 2000; 24:1353–59.
2. McCrory, M. A., P. J. Fuss, N. P. Hays, A. G. Vinken, A. S. Greenberg, and S. B. Roberts. Overeating in America: association between restaurant food consumption and body fatness in healthy adult men and women ages 19 to 80. *Obesity Research.* 1999;7(6):564–71.
3. Peregrin, T. A super-sized problem: restaurants chains piling on the food. *Journal of the American Dietetic Association.* 2001;101(6):620.
4. Zoumas-Morse, C., C. L. Rock, E. J. Sobo, and M. L. Neuhouser. Children's patterns of macronutrient intake and associations with restaurant and home eating. *Journal of the American Dietetic Association.* 2001;101(8):923–25.

CHAPTER 7

1. Borghouts, L. B., and H. A. Keizer. Exercise and insulin sensitivity: a review. *International Journal of Sports Medicine.* 2000;21(1):1–12.
2. Duncan, G. E., M. G. Perri, D. W. Theriaque, A. D. Hutson, R. H. Eckel, and P. W. Stacpoole. Exercise training, without weight loss, increases insulin sensitivity and postheparin plasma lipase activity in previously sedentary adults. *Diabetes Care.* 2003;26:557–62.

3. Eriksson, J., J. Tuominen, T. Valle, S. Sundberg, A. Sovijarvi, H. Lindholm, J. Tuomilehto, and V. Koivisto. Aerobic endurance exercise or circuit-type resistance training for individuals with impaired glucose tolerance? *Hormone and Metabolic Research.* 1998;30(1):37–41.

4. Helmrich, S. P., D. R. Ragland, and R. S. Paffenbarger. Prevention of noninsulin-dependent diabetes mellitus with physical activity. *Medicine and Science in Sports and Exercise.* 1994;26(7):824–30.

5. Hu, F. B., R. J. Sigal, J. W. Rich-Edwards, G. A. Colditz, C. G. Solomon, W. C. Willett, F. E. Speizer, and J. E. Manson. Walking compared with vigorous physical activity and risk of type 2 diabetes in women. *Journal of the American Medical Association.* 1999;282(15):1433–39.

6. Hu, F. B., M. F. Leitzmann, M. J. Stampfer, G. A. Colditz, W. C. Willett, and E. B. Rimm. Physical activity and television watching in relation to risk for type 2 diabetes mellitus in men. *Archives of Internal Medicine.* 2001;161(12):1542–48.

7. Hu, F. B., T. Y. Li, G. A. Colditz, W. C. Willett, and J. E. Manson. Television watching and other sedentary behaviors in relation to risk of obesity and type 2 diabetes mellitus in women. *Journal of the American Medical Association.* 2003;289(14):785–91.

8. Ivy, J. L. Role of exercise training in the prevention and treatment of insulin resistance and noninsulin–dependent diabetes mellitus. *Sports Medicine.* 1997;24(5):321–26.

9. Manson, J. E., D. M. Nathan, A. S. Krolewski, M. J. Stampfer, W. C. Willett, C. H. Hennekens. A prospective study of exercise and incidence of diabetes among US male physicians. *Journal of the American Medical Association.* 1992;268(1):63–67.

10. Mayer-Davis, E. J., R. D'Agostino, A. J. Karter, S. M. Haffner, M. J. Rewers, M. Saad, and R. N. Bergman. Intensity and amount of physical activity in relation to insulin sensitivity: the insulin resistance atherosclerosis study. *Journal of the American Medical Association.* 1998;279(9):669–74.

11. Ryan, A. S. Insulin resistance with aging: effects of diet and exercise. *Sports Medicine.* 2000;30(5): 327–46.

Index